Laparoscopic Surgery

Giusto Pignata
Umberto Bracale • Fabrizio Lazzara
Editors

Laparoscopic Surgery

Key Points, Operating Room Setup and Equipment

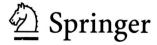 Springer

Editors
Giusto Pignata
General and Minimally Invasive Surgery
San Camillo Hospital
Trento
Italy

Fabrizio Lazzara
Department of General Surgery
Villa Igea Clinic
Acqui Terme
Alessandria
Italy

Umberto Bracale
Department of Surgical Specialities
and Nephrology
University "Federico II" of Naples
Naples
Italy

ISBN 978-3-319-24425-9   ISBN 978-3-319-24427-3   (eBook)
DOI 10.1007/978-3-319-24427-3

Library of Congress Control Number: 2015958353

Springer Cham Heidelberg New York Dordrecht London

Printed on acid-free paper

Springer International Publishing AG Switzerland is part of Springer Science+Business Media (www.springer.com)

Preface

The development of minimally invasive surgery brought to a standardization of methods, preserving as much as possible the reproducibility of surgical techniques with the use of more technologically advanced devices through courses and training schools.

The reduction of surgical risks can be achieved through a good planning and organization of the surgical team, which should have as a general rule "*who does what*".

After several training courses, I felt the need to write a book that could underline the basic rules of the surgical assessment, taking as inspiration the handbook notes of my nursing team, pointing out the position of the patient on the operating table, the equipment position, the necessary instruments, and the surgical steps.

The book aims to be a pratical handbook, of fast consultation by the medical and nursing équipe in the operating room. It could be useful to solve important problems about surgical team organization. For this reason, I use of graphic images with three-dimensional reconstruction, photos, and a checklist of surgical instruments.

I am grateful to my co-authors and to all the doctors and nurses of "*San Camillo*" Hospital in Trento who actively collaborated in the drafting of this book.

Trento, Italy   Giusto Pignata

Contents

Esophagus and Stomach

Umberto Bracale, Francesco Cabras, Ristovich Lidia,
Giovanni Merola, Plonka Elisabetta, and Giusto Pignata

The upper gastrointestinal surgery represented one of the first applications of laparoscopy. Since the early 1990s, benign esophageal disorders like gastroesophageal reflux, achalasia, or hiatal hernia became indications for the laparoscopic approach (LA) [1, 2].

During the last two decades, laparoscopy was accepted worldwide as a gold standard approach for the treatment of these diseases surpassing open surgery because of its undisputed advantages as well as less morbidity, faster recovery, and also better cosmetic results [3].

Always in the 1990s, it has been published as the first report of laparoscopic gastrointestinal resections for esophageal or gastric malignancy.

The first minimally invasive esophagectomy was reported by Cuschieri [4] in 1994. Subsequently, many reports have been published focusing on the technical aspect and feasibility of thoraco-laparoscopic esophagectomy.

With the term minimally invasive esophagectomy (MIO), it means a procedure in which both the abdominal and thoracic stages are either fully endoscopic or hand-assisted endoscopic, while hybrid MIO (HMIO) is a procedure in which one stage (abdominal or thoracic) is open and other stage is endoscopic or hand-assisted endoscopic.

U. Bracale (✉) • G. Merola
Department of Surgical Specialities and Nephrology,
University "Federico II" of Naples, Naples, Italy
e-mail: umbertobracale@gmail.com

F. Cabras
Department of General Surgery, Colo-Rectal Clinic, "Monserrato Hospital",
University of Cagliari, Monserrato, Italy

R. Lidia • P. Elisabetta • G. Pignata
Department of General Surgery, "San Camillo" Hospital, Trento, Italy
e-mail: giustopignata@gmail.com

© Springer International Publishing Switzerland 2016
G. Pignata et al. (eds.), *Laparoscopic Surgery: Key Points, Operating Room
Setup and Equipment*, DOI 10.1007/978-3-319-24427-3_1

A recent systematic review [5] analyzed the efficacy and safety including mortality, operative complications, recurrence, and quality of life of laparoscopic esophagectomy comparing to open surgery. The authors found 28 comparative studies with no randomized controlled studies (RCTs). They suggest that minimally invasive esophagectomy seems to be safe and effective as well as the open surgery. However, the quality of the researched studies is poor and with many possible bias. So they cannot conclude that minimally invasive techniques are superior to open surgery. They also suggested the best way to analyze the results of MIO in the future underlying that probably a comparative study could be adequate provided that it includes all the countless variables about patients, surgical techniques, and type of cancer.

About gastric resection for benign or malignant disease, the first laparoscopic procedure was carried out by Goh et al. in 1992 [6]. Afterward, in 1999, Azagra et al. described the first series of laparoscopically assisted gastrectomies for malignant diseases [7].

There are two types of laparoscopic procedure, the "laparoscopic assisted" (LAG) and the "totally laparoscopic" (TLG), depending if the reconstructive step is performed by a minilaparotomy (in most cases <10 cm) or fully intracorporeal. A recent meta-analysis on these two different approaches during a distal gastrectomy for an early gastric cancer (EGC) concluded that TLG can significantly reduce bleeding, time to first flatus, and rates of postoperative complications [8]. More generally, these advantages have been found frequently comparing the laparoscopic gastrectomy (LG) with the open one (OG). Another recent meta-analysis [9] demonstrated that LG decreased the frequency of analgesic administration, a shorter hospital stay, but also a longer operative times and the number of harvested lymph nodes lesser as compared to OG. These results are consistent with the conclusion of the recent Consensus Conference on Gastric Cancer of the Italian Society of Surgery [10] in which the participants suggested that a radical gastrectomy in EGC can be performed with a laparoscopic approach, while there are no data that allow to consider safe this approach for cT2 or cT3 tumors. About this issue, Hüscher et al. published the only RCT study with a 5-year follow-up [11], reporting an overall survival and disease-free survival in both groups (OG vs. TLG) of 55.7 % vs. 54.8 % and 58.9 % vs. 57.3 %, respectively. They conclude that TLG is an oncologically safe procedure.

In conclusion, it is important to recommend the use of a laparoscopy for treatment of gastric cancer only by surgeons already highly skilled in gastric surgery and in other advanced laparoscopic interventions.

We suggest to perform the first procedures during a tutoring program because it is a very complicated surgery with a long learning curve [12].

1.1   Hiatal Hernia

The bed is placed in reverse Trendelenburg position with left tilt. First operator stands between patient's legs (Figs. 1.1 and 1.5). Laparoscopic rack is placed behind patient's head.

Specific surgical drapes are used.

Laparotomic Instrument Table Must Be Always Ready for Use

Surgical Steps
1. Hernia reduction
2. Anatomical landmark recognition
3. Pars flaccida opening
4. Short gastric vessel ligation
5. Retroesophageal tunneling
6. Hiatoplasty
7. Fundusplication

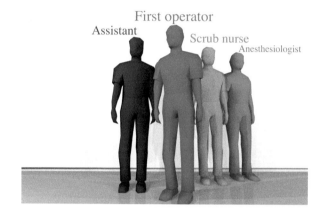

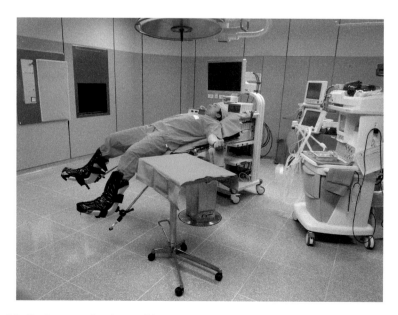

Fig. 1.1 Equipment and patient position during hiatal hernia

Instruments and Cables
- 30, 5, or 10 mm laparoscope
- Cold light source cable
- CO_2 pipe and filter
- Monopolar electrocautery
- Patient return electrode (REM)
- Sterile instrument bag
- Monopolar and bipolar electrocautery cables
- Ultrasonic dissector/radiofrequency cables
- Bladder catheterization set
- 56 Fr Maloney probe

Laparoscopic Instrument Table (Fig. 1.2)
- Sutures: 2-0 braided not absorbable suture, 0 braided absorbable suture, and skin wound closure sutures
- Surgical scalpel blade No. 23
- Laparoscopic gauzes
- Stainless surgical bowl
- Gross-Maier dressing forceps
- Two Bernhard towel forceps
- Veress needle and 10 mL syringe
- Three 10–12 mm trocars
- Two 5 mm trocars
- Needle holder
- Two tissue forceps with teeth
- Anatomical thumb forceps
- Metzenbaum scissors
- Mayo scissors
- Two Klemmer forceps
- Two Kocher forceps
- Two Backhaus forceps
- Two Farabeuf retractors
- Bipolar laparoscopic forceps
- Ultrasonic dissector/radiofrequency dissector
- Laparoscopic scissors
- Laparoscopic needle holder (2–0, 10 cm long, not absorbable braided must be ready on the instrument)
- 5–10 mm Endo Retract
- 5–10 mm clip applier
- Johann forceps without ratchet handle
- Johann forceps with ratchet handle
- 42 cm long Johann forceps without ratchet handle
- Thermos

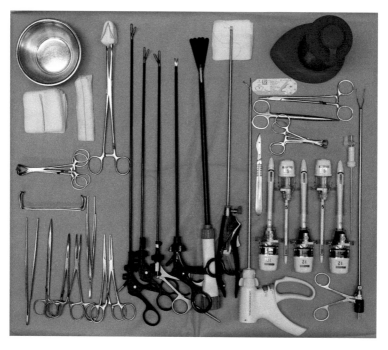

Fig. 1.2 Instrument table

1.2 Lower Esophagus Neoplastic Diseases

The bed is placed in reverse Trendelenburg position with left tilt. First operator stands between patient's legs. Laparoscopic rack is placed behind patient's head (Fig. 1.3a–d).

Specific surgical drapes are used.

Laparotomic Instrument Table Must Be Always Ready for Use

Surgical Steps
1. Anatomical landmark recognition
2. Esophageal hiatus isolation
3. Posterior mediastinum access
4. Esophageal dissection and lymphadenectomy
5. Azygos vein section (if needed)
6. Gastric tubulization

7. Kocher's maneuver
8. Cervicotomy or right thoracotomy (if needed)
9. Specimen extraction
10. Anastomosis

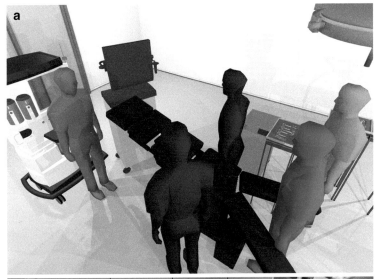

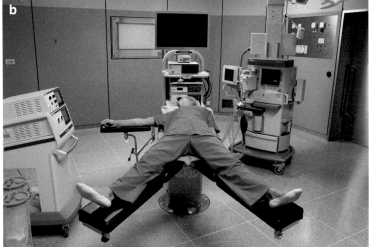

Fig. 1.3 (**a–d**) Equipment and patient position during esophagectomy

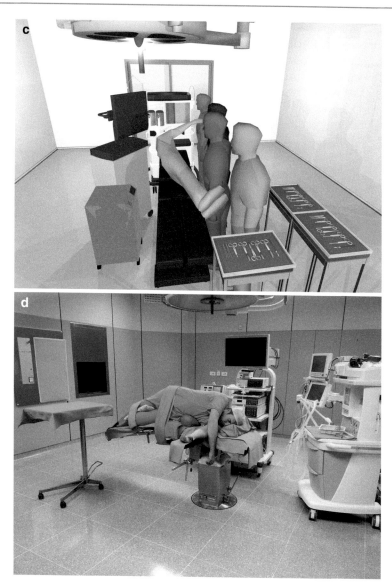

Fig. 1.3 (continued)

Instruments and Cables
- 30, 5, or 10 mm laparoscope
- Cold light source cable
- CO_2 pipe and filter
- Monopolar electrocautery
- Patient return electrode (REM)
- Sterile instrument bag

- Bipolar forceps for open surgery
- Monopolar and bipolar electrocautery cables
- Ultrasonic dissector/radiofrequency cables
- Ultrasonic dissector/radiofrequency dissector with bariatric handle and cables
- Irrigation/suction laparoscopic device
- Bladder catheterization set
- Peridural analgesic catheter and specific set

Laparoscopic Instrument Table (Fig. 1.4)
- Sutures: 2-0 braided not absorbable suture, 2-0 braided absorbable suture, and skin wound closure sutures
- Surgical scalpel blade No. 23
- Gauzes
- Laparoscopic gauzes
- Stainless surgical bowl
- Gross-Maier dressing forceps
- Two Bernhard towel forceps
- Veress needle and 10 mL syringe
- Two/one 10/12 mm trocar
- Two/three 5 mm trocars
- Needle holder
- Two tissue forceps with teeth
- Anatomical thumb forceps
- Metzenbaum scissors
- Mayo scissors
- Two Klemmer forceps
- Two Kocher forceps
- Two Backhaus forceps
- Two Farabeuf retractors
- Bipolar laparoscopic forceps
- Ultrasonic dissector/radiofrequency dissector
- Laparoscopic scissors
- Laparoscopic needle holder (2–0, 10 cm long, not absorbable braided must be ready on the instrument)
- 5–10 mm Endo Retract
- 5–10 mm clip applier
- Johann forceps without ratchet handle
- Johan forceps with ratchet handle
- 42 cm long Johan forceps without ratchet handle
- Endo GIA 45–60 mm (with cartridges)
- CEEA 25 mm
- Thermos

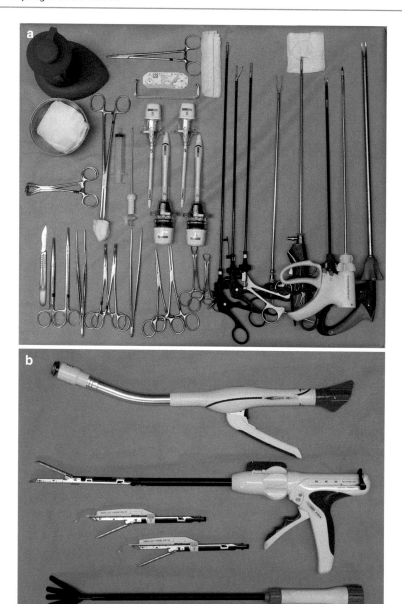

Fig. 1.4 (a–c) Instrument table

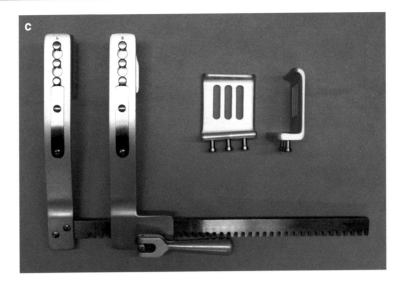

Fig. 1.4 (continued)

1.3   Gastrectomy: Gastric Resection

The bed is placed in reverse Trendelenburg position. First operator stands between patient's legs (Fig. 1.5). Laparoscopic rack is placed behind patient's head.

Specific surgical drapes are used.

Laparotomic Instrument Table Must Be Always Ready for Use

Surgical Steps
1. Anatomical landmark recognition
2. Epiploon cavity opening
3. Right gastroepiploic vessel section
4. Duodenal isolation and section
5. Pars flaccida opening
6. Hepatic pedicle lymphadenectomy and cholecystectomy (if indicated)
7. Celiac lymphadenectomy
8. Left gastric artery section
9. Small gastric vessel section
10. Gastric section (gastric resection and subtotal gastrectomy)
11. Gastric fundus and lower esophagus dissection (total gastrectomy)
12. Small intestinal loop isolation and section
13. Small bowel anastomosis
14. Gastro-digiunal anastomosis or esophagus-digiunal anastomosis

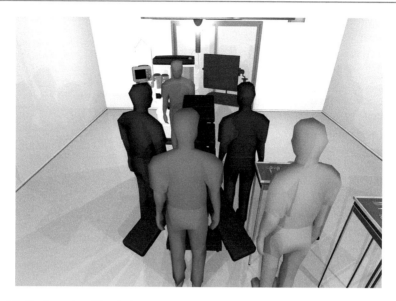

Fig. 1.5 Equipment position during gastrectomy

Instruments and Cables
- 30, 5, or 10 mm laparoscope
- Cold light source cable
- CO_2 pipe and filter
- Monopolar electrocautery
- Patient return electrode (REM)
- Two sterile instrument bags
- Bipolar forceps for open surgery
- Monopolar and bipolar electrocautery cables
- Ultrasonic dissector/radiofrequency cables
- Irrigation/suction laparoscopic device
- Bladder catheterization set

  Peridural analgesic catheter and specific set

Laparoscopic Instrument Table (Fig. 1.6)
- Sutures: 2-0 braided not absorbable suture, 2-0 braided absorbable suture, 2-0 braided absorbable suture with different colors, 3-0 barbed suture, and skin wound closure sutures
- Surgical scalpel blade No. 23
- Gauzes
- Laparoscopic gauzes
- Stainless surgical bowl
- Gross-Maier dressing forceps
- Two Bernhard towel forceps
- Veress needle and 10 mL syringe
- Three/two 10/12 mm trocars
- One/two 5 mm trocars
- Needle holders
- Two tissue forceps with teeth
- Anatomical thumb forceps
- Metzenbaum scissors
- Mayo scissors
- Two Klemmer forceps
- Two Kocher forceps
- Two Backhaus forceps
- Two Farabeuf retractors
- Bipolar laparoscopic forceps
- Ultrasonic dissector/radiofrequency dissector
- Laparoscopic scissors
- Crochet hook
- Laparoscopic needle holder (2–0, 10 cm long, not absorbable braided must be ready on the instrument)
- 5–10 mm Endo Retract
- 5–10 mm clip applier
- Johann forceps without ratchet handle
- Johan forceps with ratchet handle
- 42 cm long Johan forceps without ratchet handle
- Colored (red, white, blue) rubber loops
- Endo GIA 45/60 mm (blue cartridge for the stomach and anastomosis, white cartridge for small bowel)
- 15 mm Endobag/wound protector
- Thermos

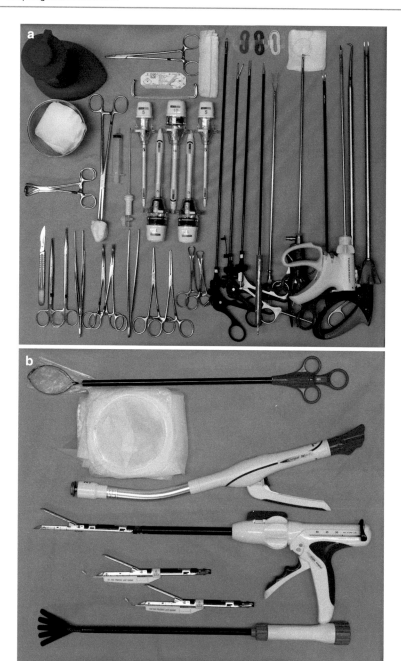

Fig. 1.6 Instrument table

References

1. Cuschieri A, Hunter J, Wolfe B, Swanstrom LL, Hutson W (1993) Multicenter prospective evaluation of laparoscopic antireflux surgery. Preliminary report. Surg Endosc 7:505–510. [PMID: 8272996 doi:10.1007/BF00316690]
2. Dallemagne B, Weerts JM, Jehaes C, Markiewicz S, Lombard R (1991) Laparoscopic Nissen fundoplication: preliminary report. Surg Laparosc Endosc 1:138–143 [PMID: 1669393]
3. Wileman SM, McCann S, Grant AM, Krukowski ZH, Bruce J (2010) Medical versus surgical management for gastrooesophageal reflux disease (GORD) in adults. Cochrane Database Syst Rev (3):CD003243. [PMID: 20238321. doi:10.1002/14651858.CD003243.pub2]
4. Cuschieri A (1994) Thoracoscopic subtotal oesophagectomy. Endosc Surg Allied Technol 2(1):21–25
5. Uttley L, Campbell F, Rhodes M, Cantrell A, Stegenga H, Lloyd-Jones M (2013) Minimally invasive oesophagectomy versus open surgery: is there an advantage? Surg Endosc 27:724–731. doi:10.1007/s00464-012-2546-3
6. Goh P, Tekant Y, Kum CK, Isaac J, Shang NS (1992) Totally intra-abdominal laparoscopic Billroth II gastrectomy. Surg Endosc 6:160. [PMID: 1386948. doi:10.1007/BF02309093]
7. Azagra JS, Georgen M, De Simone P, Ibanez-Aguire JL (1999) Minimally invasive surgery for gastric cancer. Surg Endosc 13:351–357
8. Jun G, Ping L, Jie C, Qi L, Tang D, Wang D (2013) Totally laparoscopic vs. laparoscopically assisted distal gastrectomy for gastric cancer: a meta-analysis. Hepatogastroenterology 60(126):1530–1534. doi:10.5754/hge121240
9. Deng Y et al (2015) Laparoscopy-assisted versus open distal gastrectomy for early gastric cancer: a meta-analysis based on seven randomized controlled trials. Surg Oncol 24(2):71–77. http://dx.doi.org/10.1016/j.suronc.2015.02.003
10. De Manzoni G, Baiocchi GL, Framarini M, De Giuli M, D'Ugo D et al (2014) The SIC-GIRCG 2013 Consensus Conference on Gastric Cancer. Updates Surg 66(1):1–6. doi:10.1007/s13304-014-0248-1. PMID: 24523031
11. Huscher CG, Mingoli A, Sgarzini G, Sansonetti A, Di Paola M, Recher A et al (2005) Laparoscopic versus open subtotal gastrectomy for distal gastric cancer: five-year results of a randomized prospective trial. Ann Surg 241:232
12. Bracale U, Pignata G, Lirici MM, Hüscher CG, Pugliese R, Sgroi G, Romano G, Spinoglio G, Gualtierotti M, Maglione V, Azagra S, Kanehira E, Kim JG, Song KY (2012) Laparoscopic gastrectomies for cancer: the ACOI-IHTSC national guidelines. Guideline Committee of the Italian Society of Hospital Surgeons-ACOI and Italian Hi-Tech Surgical Club-IHTSC. Minim Invasive Ther Allied Technol 21(5):313–319. doi:10.3109/13645706.2012.704877, Epub 2012 Jul 16. Review

Liver, Gallbladder, and Biliary Tree

2

Umberto Bracale, Francesco Cabras, Giovanni Merola,
Ristovich Lidia, Plonka Elisabetta, and Giusto Pignata

It is unclear who is the first surgeon to perform the first laparoscopic cholecystectomy (LC) [1]. However, Mouret reported, in March of 1987, a "laparoscopy, gynecological adhesiolysis, and cholecystectomy" for a 50-year-old woman [2].

LC represents, to date, the gold standard for gallbladder disease. It is now accepted also as a surgical procedure for acute cholecystitis when an expert surgeon performs it. There are many randomized controlled trials (RCTs) and meta-analyses, supporting the introduction of LC also for patients with acute cholecystitis founding that it is preferable early after admission [3].

There is no high scientific evidence to recommend surgery or not for patients with gallbladder polypoid lesion smaller than 10 mm [4].

The management of common bile duct stones (CBDS) includes different options.

In case of concomitant gallbladder and CBDS, endoscopic retrograde cholangio-pancreatography (ERCP) and total laparoscopic removal are equally safe provided that the latest is taken by expert laparoscopic surgeons. In case of incidental intra-operative evidence of CBDS, the best treatment choice should be laparo-endoscopic "rendezvous."

Many studies report similar outcomes between the 3-port technique and the conventional 4-port one. In the last years, the development of laparoscopic mini-instruments

U. Bracale (✉) • G. Merola
Department of Surgical Specialities and Nephrology,
University "Federico II" of Naples, Naples, Italy
e-mail: umbertobracale@gmail.com

F. Cabras
Department of General Surgery, Colo-Rectal Clinic, "Monserrato Hospital",
University of Cagliari, Cagliari, Italy

R. Lidia • P. Elisabetta • G. Pignata
Department of General Surgery, "San Camillo" Hospital, Trento, Italy
e-mail: giustopignata@gmail.com

© Springer International Publishing Switzerland 2016
G. Pignata et al. (eds.), *Laparoscopic Surgery: Key Points, Operating Room
Setup and Equipment*, DOI 10.1007/978-3-319-24427-3_2

and single-port devices led to apply more frequently these approaches. However, apart from esthetic advantages, no real benefits were reported [5].

About liver surgery, the first application of laparoscopy was reported in 1985 and consisted in drainage of an amebic liver abscess [6]. After that, the improvement and development of dedicated devices (water jet or ultrasonic dissectors and laparoscopic stapler) for the laparoscopic liver surgery permitted its application also in more complex procedures.

A significant boost in the laparoscopic liver surgery was done by the development of ultrasound devices, which overcome the lack of haptic perception.

In this way already in 1995, Hashizume et al. [7] reported the first case of laparoscopic liver resection (LR) for hepatocellular carcinoma (HCC). Thus, currently left lateral hepatectomies are performed by a mini-invasive approach in the daily practice.

Recent high-quality study confirms the feasibility and safety of LR comparing to open surgery (OS). Kim et al. [8] confirmed, in their comparative study between LR and OS for HCC (less than three-segment resection), that LR is feasible and safe in selected patients and it showed similar perioperative and long-term oncologic outcomes when compared with OR. In the same way, a meta-analysis of eight nonrandomized controlled studies [9] confirmed that LR for colorectal liver metastasis is safe and efficacious and uncompromises oncologic outcomes as compared with OLR. However, also the extended LRs (as right sided) are numerically increased, but they should only be performed in highly experienced hepatobiliary center because of their complexity.

2.1   Cholecystectomy

The bed is placed in reverse Trendelenburg position with left tilt. First operator stands between patient's legs. Laparoscopic rack is placed behind patient's head.

Specific surgical drapes are used (Figs. 2.1a, b and 2.2).

Laparotomic Instrument Table Must Be Always Ready for Use

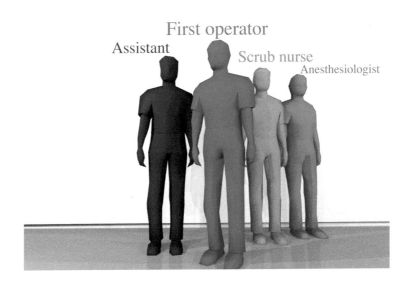

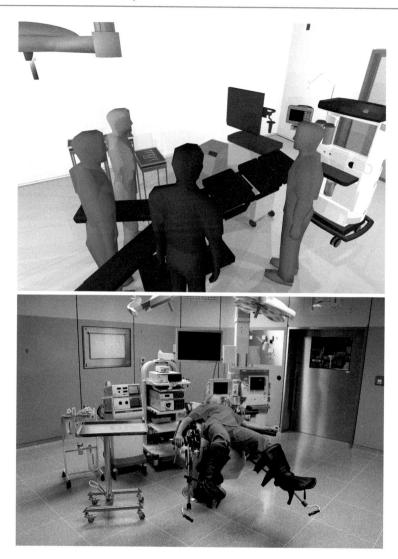

Figs. 2.1 and 2.2 Equipment and patient position

Surgical Steps
1. Adhesion dissection
2. Calot triangle opening
3. Cystic duct and artery exposition and dissection
4. Cholecystectomy
5. Specimen extraction

Laparoscopic Instrument Table (Fig. 2.3a, b)
- Sutures: 0 braided absorbable suture
- Surgical scalpel blade No. 23
- Gauzes
- Stainless surgical bowl
- Gross-Maier dressing forceps
- Two Bernhard towel forceps
- Veress needle and 10 mL syringe
- One/two 10 mm trocars
- Two/one 5 mm trocar
- Two Farabeuf retractors
- Two Backhaus forceps
- Four Kocher forceps
- Four Klemmer forceps
- Needle holder
- Foerster forceps
- Kocher ribbed gorget
- Two tissue forceps with teeth
- Metzenbaum scissors
- Mayo scissors
- Randall-Mirizzi forceps for gallstones
- Bipolar laparoscopic forceps
- Crochet hook
- Laparoscopic scissors
- Two Johann forceps or graspers
- 5–10 mm clip applier
- Thermos
- Endobag

Instruments and Cables
- 30, 5, or 10 mm laparoscope
- Cold light source cable
- CO_2 pipe and filter
- Monopolar electrocautery
- Patient return electrode (REM)
- Sterile instrument bag
- Monopolar and bipolar electrocautery cables
- Irrigation/suction laparoscopic device

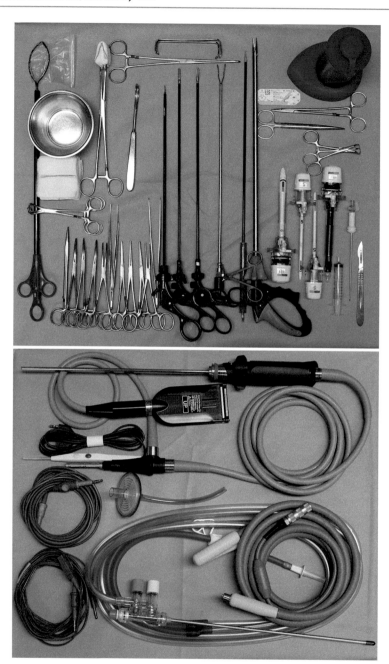

Fig. 2.3 Instrument table

2.2   Biliary Tree Surgery

The bed is placed in reverse Trendelenburg position with left tilt. First operator stands between patient's legs (Fig. 2.4). Laparoscopic rack is placed behind patient's head.

Specific surgical drapes are used.

Specific Instruments
- Coledocoscope
- Fluoroscopic C-arm machine
- Laparoscopic ultrasonography

Laparoscopic Instrument Table
- Sutures: 0 braided absorbable suture and 5-0 slowly absorbable monofilament suture
- Surgical scalpel blade No. 23
- Gauzes
- Stainless surgical bowl
- Gross-Maier dressing forceps
- Two Bernhard towel forceps
- Veress needle and 10 mL syringe
- One/two 10 mm trocars
- Two/one 5 mm trocar
- Two Farabeuf retractors
- Two Backhaus forceps
- Two Kocher forceps
- Four Klemmer forceps
- Needle holder
- Foerster forceps
- Kocher ribbed gorget
- Three tissue forceps with teeth
- Metzenbaum scissors
- Mayo scissors
- Randall-Mirizzi forceps for gallstones
- Bipolar laparoscopic forceps
- Crochet hook
- Laparoscopic scissors
- Two Johann forceps or graspers
- 5–10 mm clip applier
- Kehr probe
- Intraoperative cholangiography kit and contrast agent
- Dormia laparoscopic probe
- Fogarty catheters (various diameters)
- Thermos
- Endobag

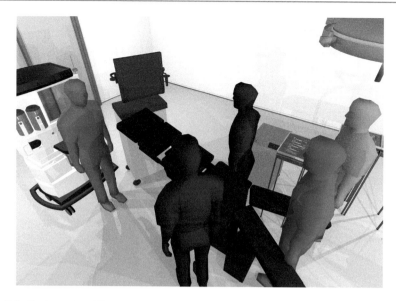

Fig. 2.4 Equipment position

Surgical Steps
1. Adhesion dissection
2. Calot triangle opening
3. Cystic duct and artery exposition and dissection
4. Cholangiography
5. Biliary stone extraction
6. Cholangiography or cholangioscopy
7. Biliary drainage or direct suture
8. Cholecystectomy
9. Specimen extraction

2.3   Hepatectomy, Liver Resection, and Wedge Liver Resection

The bed is placed in reverse Trendelenburg position. First operator stands between patient's legs. Laparoscopic rack is placed behind patient head.

Specific surgical drapes are used.

Laparotomic Instrument Table Must Be Always Ready for Use

Surgical Steps
1. Intraoperative ultrasounds
2. Hepatic pedicle isolation
3. Tourniquet placement
4. Hepatic mobilization
5. Hepatic pedicle element section
6. Hepatic section
7. Hepatic vein section
8. Specimen extraction

Specific Instruments
- Laparoscopic cavitron ultrasonic surgical aspirator (CUSA)
- Laparoscopic ultrasound probe
- Two irrigation/suction laparoscopic devices
- Bladder catheterization set
- Peridural analgesic catheter and specific set

Laparoscopic Instrument Table (Fig. 2.5 a, b)
- Sutures: 2-0 braided not absorbable suture, 2-0 braided absorbable suture, 5-0 slowly absorbable monofilament suture with vascular needle, and skin wound closure suture
- Surgical scalpel blade No. 23
- Gauzes
- Laparoscopic gauzes
- Stainless surgical bowl
- Gross-Maier dressing forceps
- Two Bernhard towel forceps
- Veress needle and 10 mL syringe
- Four/three 10–12 mm trocars

- Two/three 5 mm trocars
- Needle holder
- Two tissue forceps with teeth
- Anatomical thumb forceps
- Metzenbaum scissors
- Mayo scissors
- Two Klemmer forceps
- Two Kocher forceps
- Two Backhaus forceps
- Two Farabeuf retractors
- Bipolar laparoscopic forceps
- Laparoscopic scissors
- Crochet hook
- Laparoscopic needle holder (2–0, 10 cm long, not absorbable braided must be ready on the instrument)
- 5–10 mm Endo Retract
- 5–10 mm clip applier
- Johann forceps
- Johann forceps or graspers
- 42 cm long Johan forceps without ratchet handle
- Colored (red, white, blue) rubber loops
- Two tourniquets
- Endo GIA 45/60 mm (white cartridge)
- 15 mm Endobag/wound protector
- Thermos

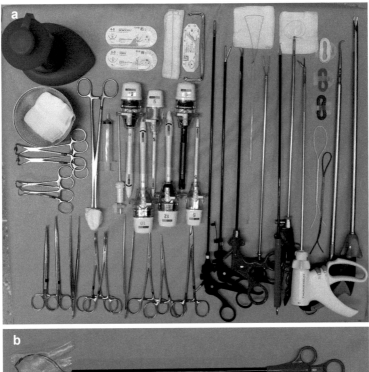

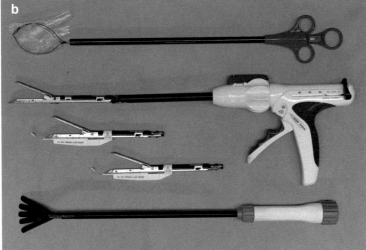

Fig. 2.5 (**a**, **b**) Instrument table

References

1. Blum CA, Adams DB (2011) Who did the first laparoscopic cholecystectomy? J Minim Access Surg 7(3):165–168. doi:10.4103/0972-9941.83506
2. Mouret P (1996) How I, developed laparoscopic cholecystectomy. Ann Acad Med Singapore 25:744–747
3. Yamashita Y, Takada T, Strasberg SM, Pitt HA, Gouma DJ, Garden OJ, Büchler MW, Gomi H, Dervenis C, Windsor JA, Kim SW, de Santibanes E, Padbury R, Chen XP, Chan AC, Fan ST, Jagannath P, Mayumi T, Yoshida M, Miura F, Tsuyuguchi T, Itoi T, Supe AN (2013) Tokyo Guideline Revision Committee. TG13 surgical management of acute cholecystitis. J Hepatobiliary Pancreat Sci 20(1):89–96. doi:10.1007/s00534-012-0567-x
4. Marangoni G, Hakeem A, Toogood GJ, Lodge JP, Prasad KR (2012) Treatment and surveillance of polypoid lesions of the gall- bladder in the United Kingdom. HPB (Oxford) 14(7):435–440
5. Agresta F, Campanile FC, Vettoretto N, Silecchia G, Bergamini C, Maida P, Lombari P, Narilli P, Marchi D, Carrara A, Esposito MG, Fiume S, Miranda G, Barlera S, Davoli M, Italian Surgical Societies Working Group on the behalf of The Italian Surgical Societies Working Group (2015) Laparoscopic cholecystectomy: consensus conference-based guidelines. Langenbecks Arch Surg 400(4):429–453. doi:10.1007/s00423-015-1300-4, Epub 2015 Apr 8
6. Salky B, Finkel S (1985) Laparoscopic drainage of amebic liver abscess. Gastrointest Endosc 31: 30–32. [PMID: 3156784. doi:10.1016/S0016-5107(85)71962-1]
7. Hashizume M, Takenaka K, Yanaga K, Ohta M, Kajiyama K, Shirabe K, Itasaka H, Nishizaki T, Sugimachi K (1995) Laparoscopic hepatic resection for hepatocellular carcinoma. Surg Endosc 9:1289–1291
8. Kim H, Suh KS, Lee KW, Yi NJ, Hong G, Suh SW, Yoo T, Park MS, Choi Y, Lee HW (2014) Long-term outcome of laparoscopic versus open liver resection for hepatocellular carcinoma: a case-controlled study with propensity score matching. Surg Endosc 28(3):950–960. doi:10.1007/s00464-013-3254-3, Epub 2013 Oct 23
9. Zhou Y, Xiao Y, Wu L, Li B, Li H (2013) Laparoscopic liver resection as a safe and efficacious alternative to open resection for colorectal liver metastasis: a meta-analysis. BMC Surg 13:44. doi:10.1186/1471-2482-13-44

Abdominal Wall Surgery

3

Jacopo Andreuccetti, Umberto Bracale, Ristovich Lidia, Lever Michele, and Giusto Pignata

Abdominal hernia diseases are the most common cause of hospitalization in Western countries. Moreover, treatment of inguinal hernias is one of the most commonly performed surgical procedures in the world [1]. Some reports have listed specific indications for laparoscopic inguinal hernia repair over open repair, including recurrent hernias, bilateral hernias, sports-oriented patients, associated pathologies, and technique request by patients [2, 3]. We described a transabdominal preperitoneal repair because we believe that this approach gives all the advantages of laparoscopic surgery. Even if TAPP hernia repair is a possible therapeutic option in scrotal and incarcerated hernia, operation time, complication rate, and frequency of recurrences are higher than in normal hernia repair [3]. A number of studies have shown that laparoscopic repair of inguinal hernias has advantages over conventional repair as reduced postoperative pain, diminished requirement for analgesics, and earlier return to work [4, 5].

Laparoscopic incisional and ventral hernia repair is preferred over open repair because of lower recurrence rates (less than 10 %), lower wound morbidity, less pain, and early return to work [6, 7]. The technique of laparoscopic repair of incisional and ventral hernia has almost been standardized, and the issues, such as the access to the abdominal cavity, mesh size, and extent of overlap, have been resolved [8–10].

Surgical treatment must be performed in an elective setting and, therefore, under ideal clinical conditions. It is essential to perform a preoperative evaluation with a

J. Andreuccetti (✉) • R. Lidia • L. Michele • G. Pignata
Department of General Surgery, "San Camillo" Hospital, Trento, Italy
e-mail: giustopignata@gmail.com

U. Bracale
Department of Surgical Specialities and Nephrology,
University "Federico II" of Naples, Naples, Italy
e-mail: umbertobracale@gmail.com

© Springer International Publishing Switzerland 2016
G. Pignata et al. (eds.), *Laparoscopic Surgery: Key Points, Operating Room
Setup and Equipment*, DOI 10.1007/978-3-319-24427-3_3

multidisciplinary approach especially in ventral and incisional hernia so as to give a correct indication for surgery centered on the patient.

Every feature of the patient should be considered and then lead to correct surgical approach. For this reason, the position of the patient reported in this book should be considered as a suggestion to the conventional cases of ventral hernia.

Nowadays, it is essential to talk about "tailored surgery." Already in 2007, Negro et al. [10] emphasized this way. He described a new therapy model based on individualized selective approach tailored to the type of hernia as well as to the characteristics of the patient. It contrasts with the past where it was one for all standard therapy.

Then laparoscopic surgery and the spread of new prosthetic materials did take off the tailored surgery.

So the surgeon plans the individual surgical approach selecting the proper technique and the right mesh for each patient.

3.1 Inguinal Hernia

The bed is placed in Trendelenburg position. The patient lies supine with arms along the body. A shoulder holder is needed. Laparoscopic rack is placed at patient's feet (Fig. 3.1).

Specific surgical drapes are used.

Laparotomic Instrument Table Must Be Always Ready for Use

Surgical Steps
1. Landmark recognition
2. Peritoneal incision
3. Preparation of a wide place for the mesh placement
4. Hernia reduction
5. Mesh placement
6. Mesh fixation
7. Peritoneal suture

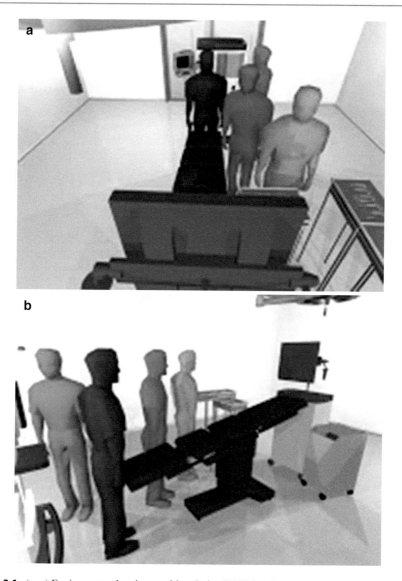

Fig. 3.1 (**a–c**) Equipment and patient position during TAPP inguinal hernia repair

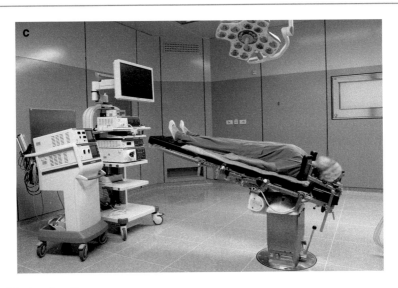

Fig. 3.1 (continued)

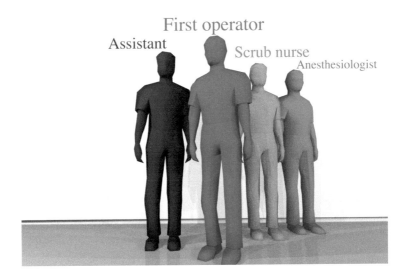

Instruments and Cables
- 30, 5, or 10 mm laparoscope
- Cold light source cable
- CO_2 pipe and filter
- Monopolar electrocautery
- Patient return electrode (REM)
- Sterile instrument bag
- Monopolar and bipolar electrocautery cables
- Bladder catheterization set

Laparoscopic Instrument Table (Fig. 3.2)
- Sutures: 0 braided absorbable suture, 3-0 barbed suture, and skin wound closure sutures
- Surgical scalpel blade No. 23
- Gauzes
- Laparoscopic gauzes
- Stainless surgical bowl
- Gross-Maier dressing forceps
- Two Bernhard towel forceps
- Veress needle and 10 mL syringe
- One 10 mm trocar
- Two 5 mm trocars
- Needle holder
- Two Backhaus forceps
- Metzenbaum scissors
- Mayo scissors
- Two tissue forceps with teeth
- Anatomical thumb forceps
- Two Kocher forceps
- Two Klemmer forceps
- Bipolar laparoscopic forceps
- Laparoscopic scissors
- Two Johann forceps without ratchet handle
- Laparoscopic needle holder
- Fibrin glue laparoscopic kit
- Thermos
- 15 cm × 10 cm mesh

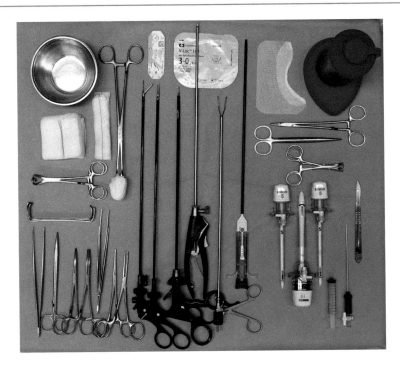

Fig. 3.2 Laparoscopic instrument table

3.2   Ventral Hernia

The bed is placed in standard position. The patient lies supine with arms along the body. Laparoscopic rack is placed on the opposite site of trocar sites (Fig. 3.3).

Specific surgical drapes are used.

Laparotomic Instrument Table Must Be Always Ready for Use

Surgical Steps
1. Adhesiolysis
2. Exposition of posterior rectal sheet
3. Hernia defect assessment
4. Mesh preparation
5. Pneumoperitoneum pressure reduction
6. Mesh fixation

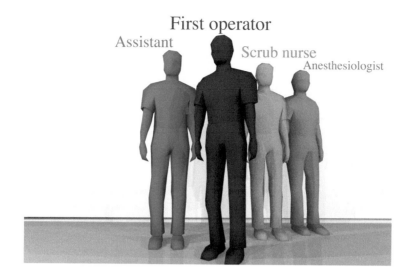

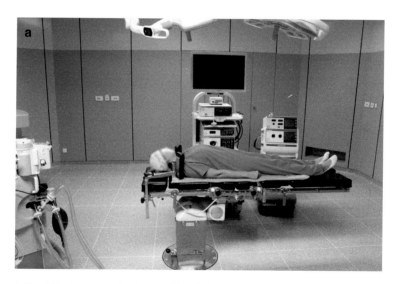

Fig. 3.3 (a–c) Equipment and patient position during ventral hernia repair

b

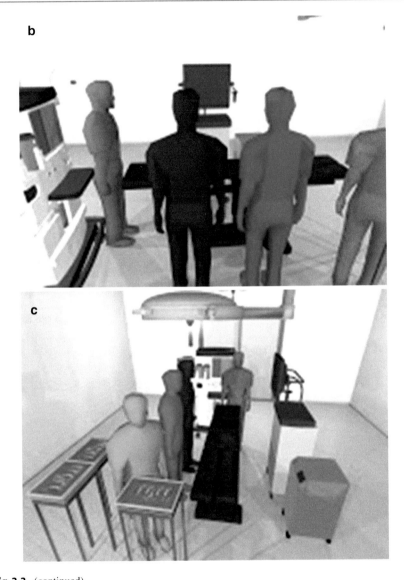

c

Fig. 3.3 (continued)

Instruments and Cables
- 30° and 5 mm laparoscope
- Cold light source cable
- CO_2 pipe and filter
- Monopolar electrocautery
- Patient return electrode (REM)
- Sterile instrument bag
- Monopolar and bipolar electrocautery cables

Laparoscopic Instrument Table (Fig. 3.4)
- Sutures: 2-0 not absorbable monofilament suture and skin wound closure sutures
- Surgical scalpel blade No. 23
- Gauzes
- Stainless surgical bowl
- Gross-Maier dressing forceps
- Two Bernhard towel forceps
- Veress needle and 10 mL syringe
- One 10 mm trocar
- Two 5 mm trocars
- Needle holder
- Two Backhaus forceps
- Two Farabeuf retractors
- Metzenbaum scissors
- Mayo scissors
- Two tissue forceps with teeth
- Two Kocher forceps
- Two Klemmer forceps
- Four mosquitos forceps
- Bipolar laparoscopic forceps
- Laparoscopic scissors
- Two Johann forceps without ratchet handle
- Spinal anesthesia needles
- Dermographic marker
- Sterile ruler
- Mesh fixation device
- Suture pass – Endo Close – Reverdin needle
- Thermos
- Intraperitoneal mesh

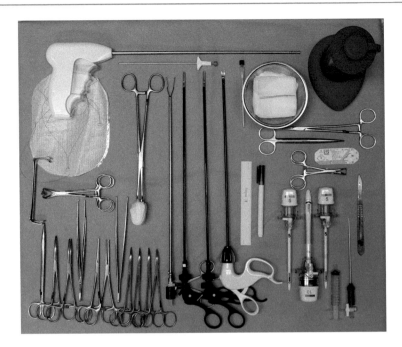

Fig. 3.4 Laparoscopic instrument table

References

1. Jenkins JT, O'Dwyer PJ (2008) Inguinal hernias. BMJ 336(7638):269–272
2. Wauschkuhn CA, Schwarz J, Boekeler U, Bittner R (2010) Laparoscopic inguinal hernia repair: gold standard in bilateral hernia repair? Results of more than 2800 patients in comparison to literature. Surg Endosc 24(12):3026–3030
3. Bittner R, Bingener-Casey J, Dietz U, Fabian M, Ferzli GS, Fortelny RH, Köckerling F, Kukleta J, Leblanc K, Lomanto D, Misra MC, Bansal VK, Morales-Conde S, Ramshaw B, Reinpold W, Rim S, Rohr M, Schrittwieser R, Simon T, Smietanski M, Stechemesser B, Timoney M, Chowbey P (2014) International Endohernia Society (IEHS). Surg Endosc 28(1):2–29. doi:10.1007/s00464-013-3170-6, Epub 2013 Oct 11
4. Bittner R, Bingener-Casey J, Dietz U, Fabian M, Ferzli GS, Fortelny RH, Köckerling F, Kukleta J, LeBlanc K, Lomanto D, Misra MC, Morales-Conde S, Ramshaw B, Reinpold W, Rim S, Rohr M, Schrittwieser R, Simon T, Smietanski M, Stechemesser B, Timoney M, Chowbey P (2014) International Endohernia Society (IEHS). Guidelines for laparoscopic treatment of ventral and incisional abdominal wall hernias (International Endohernia Society [IEHS])—Part 2. Surg Endosc. 28(2):353–379
5. Bittner R, Bingener-Casey J, Dietz U, Fabian M, Ferzli G, Fortelny R, Köckerling F, Kukleta J, LeBlanc K, Lomanto D, Misra M, Morales-Conde S, Ramshaw B, Reinpold W, Rim S, Rohr M, Schrittwieser R, Simon T, Smietanski M, Stechemesser B, Timoney M, Chowbey P (2014) International Endohernia Society (IEHS). Guidelines for laparoscopic treatment of ventral and incisional abdominal wall hernias (International Endohernia Society [IEHS])-Part III. Surg Endosc 28(2):380–404. doi:10.1007/s00464-013-3172-4. Epub 2013 Sep 17

6. Novitsky YW, Czerniach DR, Kercher KW, Kaban GK, Gallagher KA, Kelly JJ et al (2007) Advantages of laparoscopic transabdominal preperitoneal herniorrhaphy in the evaluation and management of inguinal hernias. Am J Surg 193(4):466–470

7. Fitzgibbons RJ Jr, Giobbie-Hurder A, Gibbs JO et al (2006) Watchful waiting vs repair of inguinal hernia in minimally symptomatic men: a randomized clinical trial. JAMA 295(3):285–292

8. Barbaros U, Asoglu O, Seven R et al (2007) The comparison of laparoscopic and open ventral hernia repairs: a prospective randomized study. Hernia 11:51–56 [PubMed]

9. Olmi S, Scaini A, Erba L, Croce E (2007) Use of fibrin glue (Tissucol) in laparoscopic repair of abdominal wall defects: preliminary experience. Surg Endosc 21:409–413

10. Greco VM (2014) Guida alla chirurgia Tailored dell'ernia inguinale. Page XVII Edises ISBN 978 88 7959 8217

Colon, Rectum, and Appendix

4

Francesco Cabras, Umberto Bracale, Ristovich Lidia,
Lever Michele, and Giusto Pignata

The uptake of laparoscopic colorectal surgery is increasing annually. The first laparoscopic colon resection was reported in 1991. In the United Kingdom data show that 22 % of colon resections were performed laparoscopically by 2008–2009 [1, 2].

The laparoscopic approach reduces surgical trauma and allows faster recovery from surgery, as it has been validated for other operations, such as cholecystectomy. Early reports of the outcomes of laparoscopic colorectal surgery comprised mostly nonmalignant cases, but more recently laparoscopic surgery has become widely used for colorectal cancer.

In 2010 the guidance from the UK National Institute for Health and Clinical Excellence recommended that all patients deemed suitable must be offered laparoscopic surgery even if this means onward referral to a suitably qualified surgeon [3].

The rationale for using laparoscopic surgery is that it can help minimize the trauma of access, reduce pain, and accelerate postoperative return of bowel function and general mobility. All these factors may shorten hospital stay. There are also other potential benefits including reduced adhesions and lower rates of incisional hernia.

Many surgical groups investigated the oncological adequacy during the last 20 years. The first RCT was the Colon Cancer Laparoscopic or Open Resection

F. Cabras
Department of General Surgery, Colo-Rectal Clinic, "Monserrato Hospital",
University of Cagliari, Cagliari, Italy

U. Bracale (⊠)
Department of Surgical Specialities and Nephrology,
University "Federico II" of Naples, Naples, Italy
e-mail: umbertobracale@gmail.com

R. Lidia • L. Michele • G. Pignata
Department of General Surgery, "San Camillo" Hospital, Trento, Italy
e-mail: giustopignata@gmail.com

© Springer International Publishing Switzerland 2016
G. Pignata et al. (eds.), *Laparoscopic Surgery: Key Points, Operating Room
Setup and Equipment*, DOI 10.1007/978-3-319-24427-3_4

(COLOR) Study [4, 5]. It recruited 1076 patients, operated for a colon cancer, with a median follow-up of 53 months.

The authors found a slightly higher 3-year overall survival in the open surgery group (84.2 % vs 81.8 %), but they hope the use of laparoscopic colonic resection into clinical practice.

The MRC CLASICC trial [6] was conducted in United Kingdom, and it investigated the efficacy of laparoscopy in the treatment of both colon and rectal cancer.

The researcher recruited 794 patients, and they found an overall survival, as well as the disease-free survival, comparable in both groups. However, the study showed not equally satisfying results about the circumferential resection margins for laparoscopic rectal resections.

Finally, the COLOR II trial [7, 8] investigated the oncological safety of laparoscopic rectal surgery to open surgery for rectal cancer. The authors concluded that in selected patients with rectal cancer treated by skilled surgeons, laparoscopic surgery resulted in similar safety, resection margins, and completeness of resection to that of open surgery with similar rates of locoregional recurrence and disease-free and overall survival.

In the last years, efforts to minimize the trauma of access from laparoscopic surgery have led to the development of "single-port surgery." This approach uses a single incision through which all laparoscopic instruments are passed.

A subtotal colectomy can be performed via a single 2 cm incision at the future ileostomy site, so the operation is essentially scar-free apart from the ileostomy itself [9].

It is unclear whether the benefits over conventional laparoscopy are substantial enough to justify the technical difficulties experienced by the surgeon from lack of triangulation and instrument clash [10].

4.1   Appendectomy

The bed is placed in standard position with shoulder holders. The patient lies supine with arms along the body. Laparoscopic rack is placed on the right side, slightly in the feet direction.

Specific surgical drapes are used.

Laparotomic Instrument Table Must Be Always Ready for Use.

Surgical Steps
1. Landmark recognition
2. Abdominal cavity laparoscopic exploration
3. Abdominal fluid evacuation if needed
4. Mesoappendix bipolar coagulation and section
5. Loop positioning
6. Appendectomy

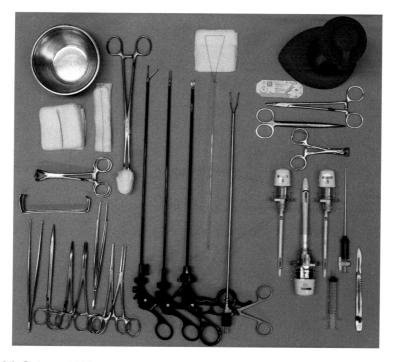

Fig. 4.1 Instrument table

Instruments and Cables
- 30° 5 mm laparoscope
- Cold light source cable
- CO_2 pipe and filter
- Monopolar electrocautery
- Patient return electrode (REM)
- Sterile instrument bag
- Monopolar and bipolar electrocautery cables

Laparoscopic Instrument Table (Fig. 4.1)
- Sutures: 0 absorbable braided suture, skin wound closure sutures
- Surgical scalpel blade No. 23
- Gauzes
- Stainless surgical bowl
- Gross-Maier dressing forceps
- 2 Bernhard towel forceps

- Veress needle and 10 mL syringe
- 1 10 mm trocars
- 2 5 mm trocars
- Needle holder
- 2 Backhaus forceps
- 2 Farabeuf retractors
- Metzenbaum scissors
- Mayo scissors
- 2 tissue forceps with teeth
- Anatomical thumb forceps
- 2 Kocher forceps
- 2 Klemmer forceps
- 2 endoloop (2-0 absorbable braided)
- Bipolar laparoscopic forceps
- Laparoscopic scissors
- 2 Johann forceps without ratchet handle
- Thermos

4.2   Right Colectomy

The bed is placed in standard position with shoulder holders. The patient lies supine with left arm along the body. Laparoscopic rack is placed on the right side (Fig. 4.2).

Specific surgical drapes are used.

Laparotomic Instrument Table Must Be Always Ready for Use.

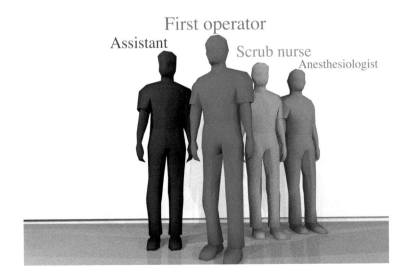

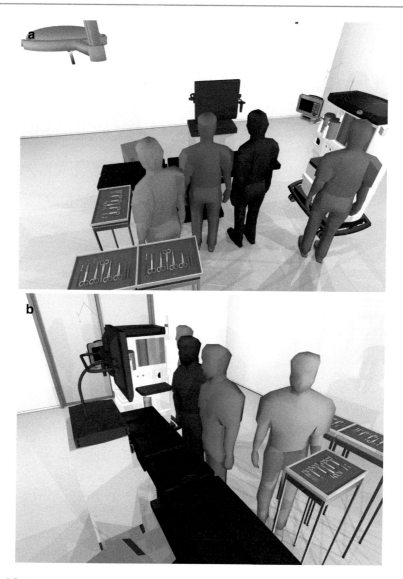

Fig. 4.2 (**a–c**) Equipe and patient position during appendectomy and right colectomy

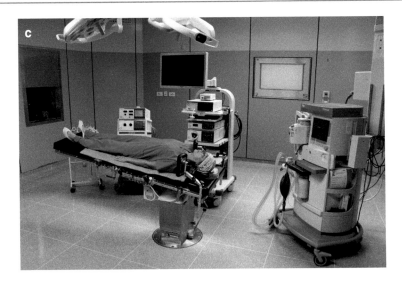

Fig. 4.2 (continued)

Surgical Steps
1. Landmark recognition
2. Colic vessel isolation and section
3. Transverse colon mobilization and isolation
4. Ileus mobilization and isolation
5. Intracorporeal ileocolic anastomosis
6. Specimen extraction with Pfannenstiel incision

Instruments and Cables
- 30° 5/10 mm laparoscope
- Cold light source cable
- CO_2 pipe and filter
- Monopolar electrocautery
- Patient return electrode (REM)
- 2 sterile instrument bags
- Bipolar laparotomic forceps
- Monopolar and bipolar electrocautery cables
- Ultrasonic dissector/radio-frequency cables
- Irrigation/suction laparoscopic device
- Bladder catheterization set

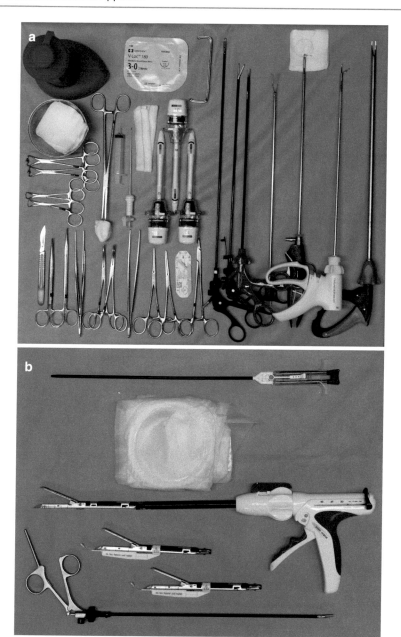

Fig. 4.3 (**a**, **b**) Instrument table

Laparoscopic Instrument Table (Fig. 4.3 a, b)
- Sutures: 2-0 not absorbable braided suture, 3-0 slowly absorbable barbed suture, 0 braided absorbable suture, skin wound closure sutures
- Surgical scalpel blade No. 23
- Gauzes
- Laparoscopic gauzes
- Stainless surgical bowl
- Gross-Maier dressing forceps
- 2 Bernhard towel forceps
- Veress needle and 10 mL syringe
- 3 10/12 mm trocars
- 0/1 5 mm trocars
- Needle holders (different dimensions)
- 2 tissue forceps with teeth
- 2 anatomical thumb forceps
- Metzenbaum scissors
- Mayo scissors
- 2 Klemmer forceps
- 2 Kocher forceps
- 2 Backhaus forceps
- 2 Farabeuf retractors
- Bipolar laparoscopic forceps
- Laparoscopic scissors
- Laparoscopic needle holder (2-0, 10 cm long, not absorbable braided must be ready on the instrument)
- 5–10 mm clip applier
- Ultrasonic/radio-frequency dissector
- 2 Johann forceps without ratchet handle
- Johann forceps with ratchet handle
- Endo-GIA 45 mm (white cartridge for ileus, blue cartridge for colon and anastomosis)
- Fibrin glue laparoscopic kit
- 15 mm endobag/wound protector
- Thermos

4.3   Left Colectomy and Rectal Resection

The bed is placed in Lloyd-Davies position with shoulder holders. The patient lies supine with right arm along the body. Laparoscopic rack is placed on the left side (Fig. 4.4).

Specific surgical drapes are used.

Laparotomic Instrument Table Must Be Always Ready for Use.

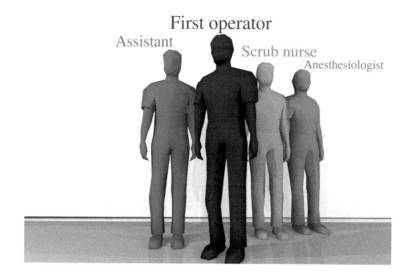

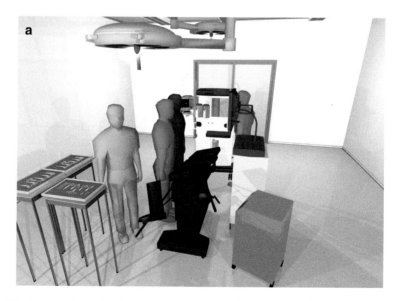

Fig. 4.4 (a–c) Equipe and patient position during left colectomy or rectal resection

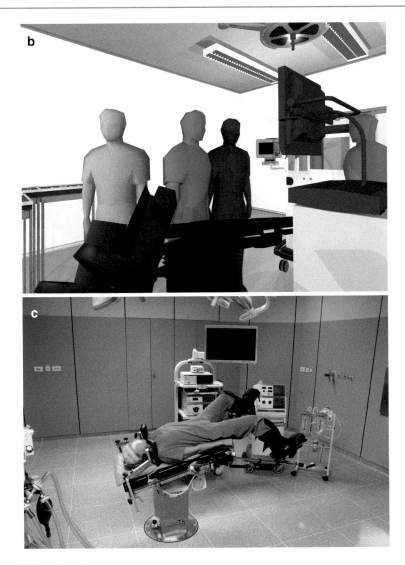

Fig. 4.4 (continued)

Surgical Steps
1. Landmark recognition
2. Left colic angle isolation
3. Vascular isolation
4. Left colon isolation
5. Vascular section
6. Colic section
7. Specimen exteriorization

8. Specimen section and extraction
9. CEEA anvil positioning
10. Colorectal anastomosis
11. Anastomosis check

Instruments and Cables
- 30° 5/10 mm laparoscope
- Cold light source cable
- CO_2 pipe and filter
- Monopolar electrocautery
- Patient return electrode (REM)
- 2 sterile instrument bags
- Bipolar laparotomic forceps
- Monopolar and bipolar electrocautery cables
- Ultrasonic/radio-frequency cables
- Irrigation/suction laparoscopic device
- Bladder catheterization set
- Peridural analgesic catheter and specific set

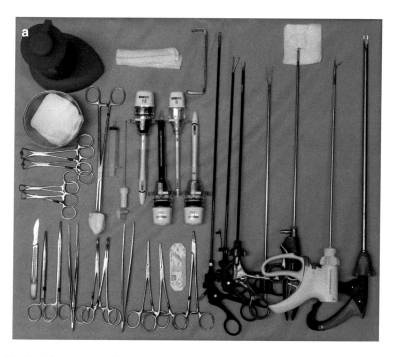

Fig. 4.5 (**a–c**) Instrument table

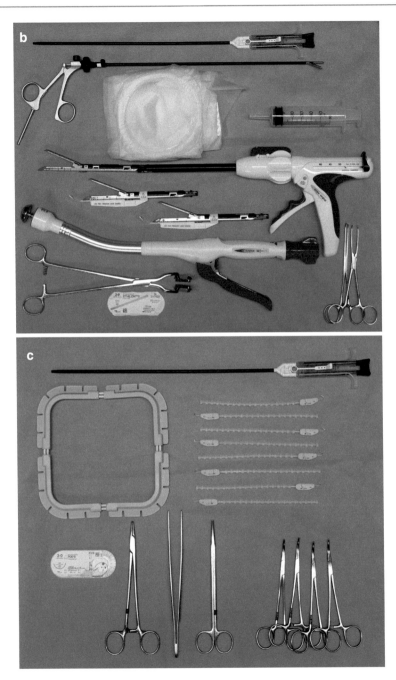

Fig. 4.5 (continued)

Laparoscopic Instrument Table (Fig. 4.5 a–c)
- Sutures: 2-0 not absorbable braided suture, 2-0 monofilament suture with double straight needle, skin wound closure sutures
- Surgical scalpel blade No. 23
- Gauzes
- Laparoscopic gauzes
- Stainless surgical bowl
- Gross-Maier dressing forceps
- 2 Bernhard towel forceps
- Veress needle and 10 mL syringe
- 3 10/12 mm trocars
- 1 5 mm trocars
- 1 needle holder
- 2 tissue forceps with teeth
- 2 anatomical thumb forceps
- Metzenbaum scissors
- Mayo scissors
- 2 Klemmer forceps
- 2 Kocher forceps
- 2 Farabeuf retractors
- 2 Hellis forceps
- Purse string
- Bipolar laparoscopic forceps
- Laparoscopic scissors
- Laparoscopic needle holder (2-0, 10 cm long, not absorbable braided must be ready on the instrument)
- 5–10 mm clip applier
- Ultrasonic/radio-frequency dissector
- Johann forceps without ratchet handle
- 42 cm long Johan forceps without ratchet handle
- Endo-GIA 45 mm (blue and/or green cartridges)
- CEEA 29 mm
- 60 mL syringe
- Fibrin glue laparoscopic kit
- Wound protector
- Lone star retractor
- Thermos

References

1. Nachmany I, Pencovich N, Zohar N, Ben-Yehuda A, Binyamin C, Goykhman Y, Lubezky N, Nakache R, Klausner JM (2015) Laparoscopic versus open liver resection for metastatic colorectal cancer. Eur J Surg Oncol. pii: S0748-7983(15)00781-7. doi: 10.1016/j. ejso.2015.09.014.
2. Jacobs M, Verdeja JC, Goldstein HS (1991) Minimally invasive colon resection (laparoscopic colectomy). Surg Laparosc Endosc 1:144–150
3. National Institute for Health and Clinical Excellence (2006) Laparoscopic surgery for colorectal cancer. https://www.nice.org.uk/guidance/ta105
4. Clinical Outcomes of Surgical Therapy Study Group (2004) A comparison of laparoscopically assisted and open colectomy for colon cancer. N Engl J Med 350:2050–2059. [PMID: 15141043. doi:10.1056/NEJMoa032651] 118
5. Buunen M, Veldkamp R, Hop WC, Kuhry E, Jeekel J, Haglind E, Påhlman L, Cuesta MA, Msika S, Morino M, Lacy A, Bonjer HJ (2009) Survival after laparoscopic surgery versus open surgery for colon cancer: long-term outcome of a randomised clinical trial. Lancet Oncol 10:44–52. [PMID: 19071061. doi:10.1016/S1470-2045(08)70310-3]
6. Jayne DG, Guillou PJ, Thorpe H, Quirke P, Copeland J, Smith AM, Heath RM, Brown JM (2007) Randomized trial of laparoscopic-assisted resection of colorectal carcinoma: 3-year results of the UK MRC CLASICC Trial Group. J Clin Oncol 25:3061–3068. [PMID: 17634484. doi:10.1200/JCO.2006.09.7758]
7. van der Pas MH, Haglind E, Cuesta MA, Fürst A, Lacy AM, Hop WC, Bonjer HJ (2013) Laparoscopic versus open surgery for rectal cancer (COLOR II): short-term outcomes of a randomised, phase 3 trial. Lancet Oncol 14: 210–218. [PMID: 23395398. doi:10.1016/ S1470-2045(13)70016-0]
8. Bonjer HJ, Deijen CL, Abis GA, Cuesta MA, van der Pas MH, de Lange-de Klerk ES, Lacy AM, Bemelman WA, Andersson J, Angenete E, Rosenberg J, Fuerst A, Haglind E, COLOR II Study Group (2015) A randomized trial of laparoscopic versus open surgery for rectal cancer. N Engl J Med 372(14):1324–1332. doi:10.1056/NEJMoa1414882
9. Cahill RA, Lindsey I, Jones O, Guy R, Mortensen N, Cunningham C (2010) Single-port laparoscopic total colectomy for medically uncontrolled colitis. Dis Colon Rectum 53:1143–1147
10. Bracale U, Melillo P, Lazzara F, Andreuccetti J, Stabilini C, Corcione F, Pignata G (2015) Single-access laparoscopic rectal resection versus the multiport technique: a retrospective study with cost analysis. Surg Innov 22(1):46–53. doi:10.1177/1553350614529668, Epub 2014 Apr 14

Kidney, Adrenal Gland, Ureter, and Varicocele

5

Fabrizio Lazzara, Jacopo Andreuccetti, Lidija Ristovich, Elisabetta Plonka, and Giusto Pignata

From early nephrectomies carried out in 1990s, radical nephrectomy nowadays reaches a high diffusion between surgeons and finds specific indications. In 2014 *The European Association of Urology* built a Renal Cell Carcinoma Guideline Panel and created evidence-based recommendations [1]. Laparoscopic radical nephrectomy has the same oncological outcomes of open approach, and it is the gold standard for T2 renal tumors. It allows shorter hospital stay and less use of analgesics, so it is preferable than the open approach for the lower morbidity rate. Two laparoscopic approaches are described: transperitoneal and retroperitoneal. There are few differences, mostly concerning the easier hilar structure approach with retroperitoneal approach. We describe the transabdominal one because of the more usual landmark identification for a general surgeon.

For less extended renal carcinoma (T1a; T1b), partial nephrectomy is preferred, both with open and laparoscopic approach. There is some debate about the best approach for larger tumor (T3), but a laparoscopic approach seems to be safe in experienced hands [2].

In the field of laparoscopic urologic surgery, there is a growing consensus for reconstructive procedures [3]. A general surgeon sometimes needs to work in direct contact with the ureter, for example, during colorectal resections and gynecological procedures; so there could be the need to perform ureter resections and ureteral bladder reimplantation. The first laparoscopic reimplantation was described by Nezhat et al. in 1992 [4]. Up to now, open surgery is still widely chosen because this kind of laparoscopic surgery is technically demanding even for urologists.

F. Lazzara (✉)
Department of General Surgery, Villa Igea Clinic, Acqui Terme, Alessandria, Italy
e-mail: f.lazzara@gmail.com

J. Andreuccetti • L. Ristovich • E. Plonka • G. Pignata
Department of General Surgery, "San Camillo" Hospital, Trento, Italy
e-mail: giustopignata@gmail.com

© Springer International Publishing Switzerland 2016
G. Pignata et al. (eds.), *Laparoscopic Surgery: Key Points, Operating Room Setup and Equipment*, DOI 10.1007/978-3-319-24427-3_5

Laparoscopic approach is useful for the image magnification and the easier structure identification.

Laparoscopic adrenalectomy is indicated for benign neoplasm smaller than 6 cm even if it is described as safe and feasible even in bigger lesions and for malignancies without radiological signs of local tissue infiltration [5]. Gagner described the first cases in 1992 [6]. Like in other procedures for retroperitoneal organs, two approaches are described: an anterior or lateral transperitoneal approach and a retroperitoneal approach. We describe an anterior transperitoneal approach, which is more familiar for a general surgeon.

Varicocele laparoscopic treatment is a basic procedure mostly useful for children and young patient in which local anesthesia is not an option, or in case of concomitant laparoscopic procedures. It offers the advantage of bilateral treatment and its results are similar to open techniques [7]. We describe this technique because it is a very basic laparoscopic procedure but gives to the surgeon an approach to an anatomical region, which is the site of more advanced procedures like laparoscopic transabdominal preperitoneal hernia repair.

5.1 Nephrectomy and Adrenalectomy

The bed is placed in standard position. The patient lies on the opposite side of the kidney with the arm holder on the same side and opposite arm left free. A pillow must be placed between legs, with the inferior leg slightly flexed. Ankle strap and a lateral holder on the gluteus muscle are used. Laparoscopic rack is placed at the back of the patient (Fig. 5.1a, b).

Surgical Steps in Nephrectomy
1. Landmark recognition
2. Colon mobilization
3. Renal vein isolation
4. Renal artery isolation and section
5. Renal vein section
6. Ureter and gonadic vessels
7. Nephrectomy (adrenalectomy if needed)

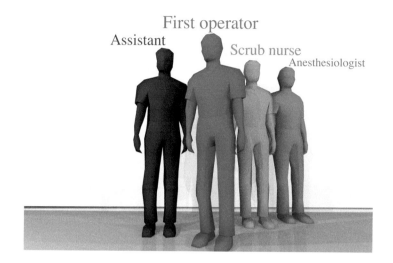

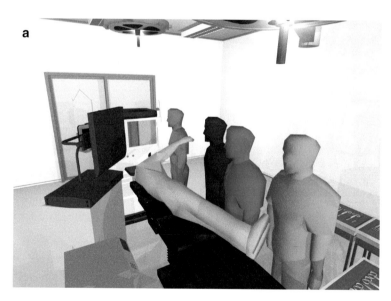

Fig. 5.1 (**a**, **b**) Equipment and patient position during right and left nephrectomy/adrenalectomy

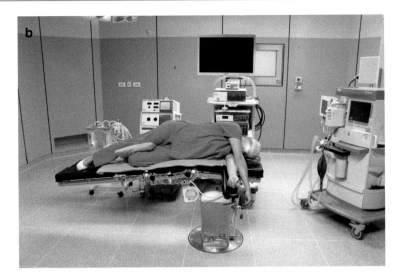

Fig. 5.1 (continued)

Surgical Steps (Left Adrenal Gland)
1. Landmark recognition
2. Colon mobilization
3. Splenopancreatic mobilization
4. Renal vein isolation
5. Adrenal vein isolation and section
6. Left adrenalectomy

Surgical Steps (Right Adrenal Gland)
1. Landmark recognition
2. Colon mobilization
3. Caval vein exposition
4. Adrenal vein isolation and section
5. Right adrenalectomy

5.2   Equipment in Nephrectomy and Adrenalectomy

Instruments and Cables
Specific surgical drapes are used.

- 30 and 5/10 mm laparoscope
- Cold light source cable

- CO_2 pipe and filter
- Monopolar electrocautery
- Patient return electrode (REM)
- Two sterile instrument bags
- Bipolar laparotomic forceps
- Monopolar and bipolar electrocautery cables
- Ultrasonic dissector or radiofrequency cables
- Irrigation/suction laparoscopic device
- Bladder catheterization set
- Peridural analgesic catheter and specific set

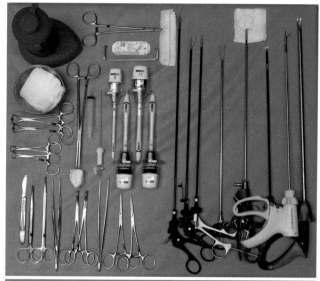

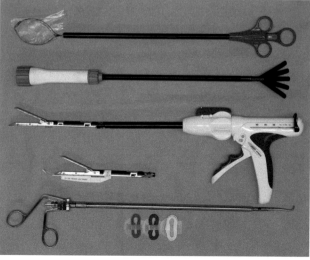

Fig. 5.2 Instrument table

Laparoscopic Instrument Table (Fig. 5.2)
- Sutures: 2-0 absorbable braided suture, 5-0 monofilament not absorbable, one suture with vascular needle, one braided absorbable suture, and one skin wound closure sutures
- Surgical scalpel blade No. 23
- Gauzes
- Laparoscopic gauzes
- Stainless surgical bowl
- Gross-Maier dressing forceps
- Two Bernhard towel forceps
- Veress needle and 10 mL syringe
- Two 10/12 mm trocars
- Two 5 mm trocars
- Needle holder
- Two tissue forceps with teeth
- Metzenbaum scissors
- Mayo scissors
- Two Klemmer forceps
- Two Kocher forceps
- Two Backhaus forceps
- Two Farabeuf retractors
- Bipolar laparoscopic forceps
- Ultrasonic dissector
- Radiofrequency dissector
- Laparoscopic scissors
- Laparoscopic needle holder (2–0, 10 cm long, not absorbable braided must be ready on the instrument)
- 5–10 mm Endo Retract
- 10 mm clip applier
- Two Johann forceps without ratchet handle
- 42 cm long Johan forceps without ratchet handle
- Colored (red, white, blue) rubber loops
- Endo GIA 45 mm (vascular cartridge)
- Laparoscopic 90° forceps with rounded tip
- 15 mm Endobag/wound protector
- Thermos

5.3   Ureteral Reimplantation and Varicocelectomy

The bed is placed in Trendelenburg position with leg holders. The patient lies supine with both arms along the body. Laparoscopic rack is placed on the same side of the ureter. (Fig. 5.3a, b)

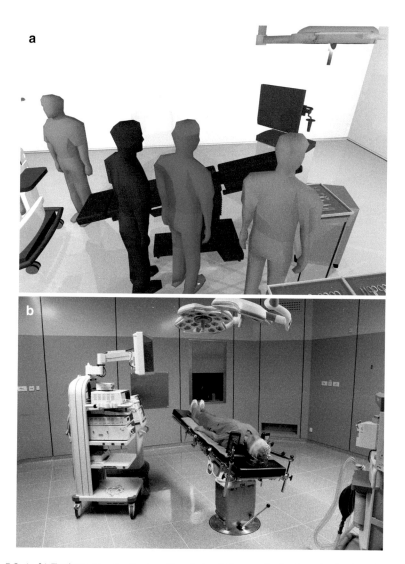

Fig. 5.3 (**a**, **b**) Equipment and patient position during left ureteral reimplantation/varicocelectomy

Surgical Steps: Ureteral Reimplantation
1. Landmark recognition
2. Colon mobilization if needed
3. Isolation and section of ureter
4. Bladder filling
5. Bladder fixation to the psoas muscle
6. Ureteral catheterization and uretrovescical anastomosis

Surgical Steps: Varicocelectomy
1. Landmark recognition
2. Peritoneal incision
3. Gonadic vein isolation
4. Clip positioning and section

5.4 Equipment in Ureteral Reimplantation

Instruments and Cables
Specific surgical drapes are used.

- 30 and 5/10 mm laparoscope.
- Cold light source cable.
- CO_2 pipe and filter.
- Monopolar electrocautery.
- Patient return electrode (REM).
- Two sterile instrument bags.
- Bipolar laparotomic forceps.
- Monopolar and bipolar electrocautery cables.
- Irrigation/suction laparoscopic device.
- Bladder catheterization set.

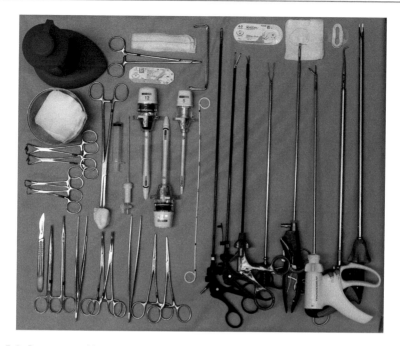

Fig. 5.4 Instrument table

Laparoscopic Instrument Table (Fig. 5.4)
- Sutures: 2-0 not absorbable braided suture, 2-0 not absorbable braided suture, 1 braided absorbable suture, 3-0 barbed suture, and skin wound closure sutures
- Surgical scalpel blade No. 23
- Gauzes
- Laparoscopic gauzes
- Stainless surgical bowl
- Gross-Maier dressing forceps
- Two Bernhard towel forceps
- Veress needle and 10 mL syringe
- Two 10/12 mm trocars
- One 5 mm trocar
- Needle holder
- Needle holders (different dimensions)

- Two tissue forceps with teeth
- Anatomical thumb forceps
- Metzenbaum scissors
- Mayo scissors
- Two Klemmer forceps
- Two Kocher forceps
- Two Backhaus forceps
- Two Farabeuf retractors
- Bipolar laparoscopic forceps
- Laparoscopic scissors
- Laparoscopic needle holder (2–0, 10 cm long, not absorbable must be ready on the instrument)
- 5/10 mm clip applier
- Two Johann forceps without ratchet handle
- 42 cm long Johann forceps without ratchet handle
- Colored (yellow or white) rubber loops
- Laparoscopic 90° forceps with rounded tip
- Double J ureteral catheter
- Thermos

5.5   Equipment in Varicocelectomy

Instruments and Cables
- 30 and 5 mm laparoscope
- Cold light source cable
- CO_2 pipe and filter
- Monopolar electrocautery
- Patient return electrode (REM)
- Sterile instrument bag
- Monopolar and bipolar electrocautery cables

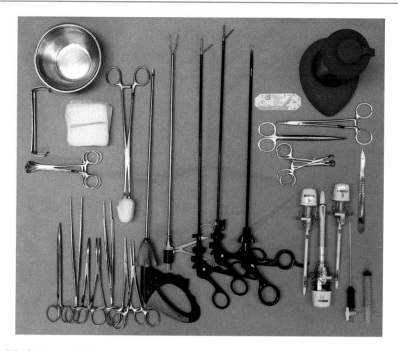

Fig. 5.5 Instrument table

Laparoscopic Instrument Table (Fig. 5.5)
- Sutures: 0 braided absorbable suture and skin wound closure sutures
- Surgical scalpel blade No. 23
- Gauzes
- Laparoscopic gauzes
- Stainless surgical bowl
- Gross-Maier dressing forceps
- Two Bernhard towel forceps
- Veress needle and 10 mL syringe
- One 10 mm trocars
- Two 5 mm trocars
- Needle holder
- Two Backhaus forceps

- Metzenbaum scissors
- Mayo scissors
- Two tissue forceps with teeth
- Two Kocher forceps
- Two Farabeuf retractors
- Two Klemmer forceps
- Bipolar laparoscopic forceps
- Laparoscopic scissors
- Two Johann forceps without ratchet handle
- 5–10 mm clip applier
- Thermos

References

1. Ljungberg B, Bensalah K, Canfield S, Dabestani S, Hofmann F, Hora M, Kuczyk MA, Lam T, Marconi L, Merseburger AS, Mulders P, Powles T, Staehler M, Volpe A, Bex A (2015) EAU guidelines on renal cell carcinoma: 2014 update. Eur Urol 67(5):913–924.
2. Stewart GD, Ang WJ, Laird A, Tolley DA, Riddick AC, McNeill SA (2012) The operative safety and oncological outcomes of laparoscopic nephrectomy for T3 renal cell cancer. BJU Int 110(6):884–890.
3. Rassweiler J, Pini G, Gözen AS, Klein J, Teber D (2010) Role of laparoscopy in reconstructive surgery. Curr Opin Urol 20(6):471–482.
4. Nezhat C, Nezhat F (1992) Laparoscopic repair of ureter resected during operative laparos-copy. Obstet Gynecol 80(3 Pt 2):543–544.
5. Ramacciato G, Mercantini P, La Torre M, Di Benedetto F, Ercolani G, Ravaioli M, Piccoli M, Melotti G (2008) Is laparoscopic adrenalectomy safe and effective for adrenal masses larger than 7 cm? Surg Endosc 22(2):516–521.
6. Gagner M, Lacroix A, Bolté E (1992) Laparoscopic adrenalectomy in Cushing's syndrome and pheochromocytoma. N Engl J Med 327(14):1033.
7. Borruto FA, Impellizzeri P, Antonuccio P, Finocchiaro A, Scalfari G, Arena F, Esposito C, Romeo C (2010) Laparoscopic vs open varicocelectomy in children and adolescents: review of the recent literature and meta-analysis. J Pediatr Surg 45(12):2464–2469.

Spleen and Pancreas

6

Fabrizio Lazzara, Jacopo Andreuccetti, Ristovich Lidia, Plonka Elisabetta, and Giusto Pignata

Splenectomy is a surgical treatment for hematologic diseases like platelet dysfunctions and autoimmune anemia; it is used for lymphoma stadiation and for splenic neoplasms. Laparoscopic surgery for spleen diseases is widely adopted among surgeons as a safe and feasible alternative to open surgery. Laparoscopic post-traumatic urgency surgery is increasing diffusion and it has specific indications. In selected centers and among experienced laparoscopic surgeons, it is chosen for the treatment of hemoperitoneum for spleen rupture, and it allows also reduction of unnecessary diagnostic laparotomies [1].

Laparoscopic splenectomy offers benefits for patients like decreased mortality, postoperative respiratory morbidity, incisional hernia, and sepsis. It is also associated with faster recovery and shorter hospital stay and fewer need for intraoperative transfusions [2]. When the integrity of the specimen is not a major issue, like in benign splenic diseases or hypersplenism, wounds and scars can be further reduced. This is done thanks to the use of specimen morcellation and reduced access laparoscopic surgery. In this field, the robotic surgery could find a good application [3].

The first laparoscopic splenectomy was reported in 1991 by Delaitre and Maignein [4]. In few years, the first laparoscopic splenectomy for splenomegaly was carried out by Poulin and Thibault [5]. The evolution of the technique and the use of laparoscopic advanced cutting and sealing devices allow now shorter operative time and improve safety. In 2007, the *European Association for Endoscopic Surgery* organized a consensus conference to create practical guidelines in laparoscopic splenectomy [6]. The laparoscopic approach was described as preferable to the open approach for most indications.

F. Lazzara (✉)
Department of General Surgery, Villa Igea Clinic, Acqui Terme, Alessandria, Italy
e-mail: f.lazzara@gmail.com

J. Andreuccetti • R. Lidia • P. Elisabetta • G. Pignata
Department of General Surgery, "San Camillo" Hospital, Trento, Italy
e-mail: giustopignata@gmail.com

© Springer International Publishing Switzerland 2016
G. Pignata et al. (eds.), *Laparoscopic Surgery: Key Points, Operating Room Setup and Equipment*, DOI 10.1007/978-3-319-24427-3_6

Similarly, laparoscopic surgery is getting relevance in pancreas surgery. Pancreatic resections are difficult operations because of the retroperitoneal location of the gland, surrounded by big vascular structures, and they are characterized by high morbidity and mortality rate.

Laparoscopic right-sided pancreatic resections are uncommon procedures proposed in highly specialized mini-invasive surgical centers. Left-sided pancreatic resections are instead getting popular and are showing benefits compared to open approach.

Laparoscopic left pancreas resections, associated or not with splenectomy, are described as safe procedures [7], but in this field of research randomized controlled studies are lacking. These procedures can offer shorter operative time and shorter hospital stay, less blood loss, less perioperative mortality and morbidity, less pancreatic fistulas, less abscesses, less bleeding, and less wound infections compared to standard open approaches.

In selected patient with small lesions and low body mass index, distal pancreatectomy has been feasible with a single access laparoscopic surgery, offering a safe alternative with the aim of reducing invasiveness [8, 9].

6.1   Splenectomy

The bed is placed in reverse Trendelenburg position. Patient lies on the right side. Right arm holder is needed, and left arm is left free. A pillow must be placed between legs, with the inferior leg slightly flexed. Ankle strap, and a lateral holder on the gluteus muscle are used. Laparoscopic rack is placed at the back of the patient (Fig 6.1).

Specific surgical drapes are used.

Laparotomic Instrument Table Must Be Always Ready for Use

Surgical Steps
1. Landmark recognition
2. Left colic angle mobilization
3. Short gastric vessel section
4. Isolation and clip application on splenic artery
5. Isolation and section of splenic vessels
6. Clip removal
7. Splenectomy
8. Specimen extraction on Pfannensteil incision

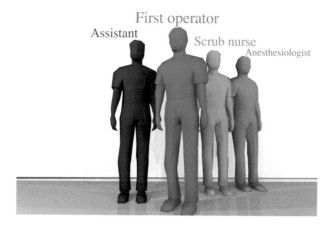

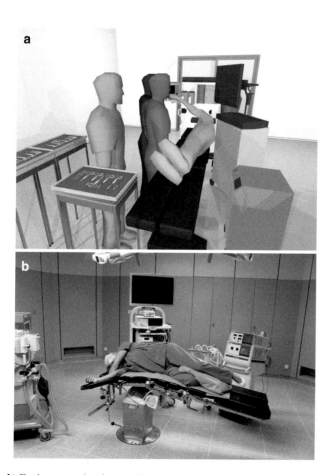

Fig. 6.1 (**a**, **b**) Equipment and patient position during splenectomy

Instruments and Cables
- 30 and 5/10 mm laparoscope
- Cold light source cable
- CO_2 pipe and filter
- Monopolar electrocautery
- Patient return electrode (REM)
- Sterile instrument bags
- Bipolar laparotomic forceps
- Monopolar and bipolar electrocautery cables
- Ultrasonic dissector/radiofrequency cables
- Irrigation/suction laparoscopic device
- Bladder catheterization set

Laparoscopic Instrument Table (Figs. 6.2 and 6.3)
- Sutures: 2-0 absorbable braided suture and skin wound closure sutures
- Surgical scalpel blade No. 23
- Gauzes
- Laparoscopic gauzes
- Stainless surgical bowl
- Gross-Maier dressing forceps
- Two Bernhard towel forceps
- Veress needle and 10 mL syringe
- Two/three 10/12 mm trocars
- One/two 5 mm trocars
- Needle holder
- Two tissue forceps with teeth
- Metzenbaum scissors
- Mayo scissors
- Two Klemmer forceps
- Two Kocher forceps
- Two Backhaus forceps
- Two Farabeuf retractors
- Bipolar laparoscopic forceps
- Ultrasonic dissector/radiofrequency dissector
- Laparoscopic scissors
- Laparoscopic needle holder (2–0, 10 cm long, not absorbable braided must be ready on the instrument)
- 5–10 mm clip applier
- Two Johann forceps without ratchet handle
- 56 cm long Johan forceps without ratchet handle
- Endo GIA 45 mm (vascular cartridge)
- Laparoscopic 90° forceps with rounded tip
- 15 mm Endobag
- Thermos

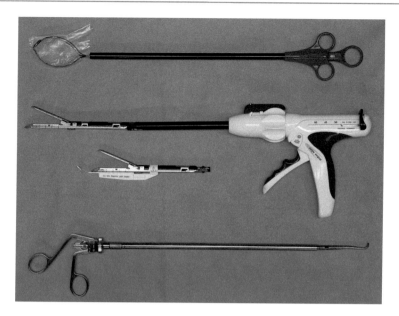

Fig. 6.2 Laparoscopic instrument table

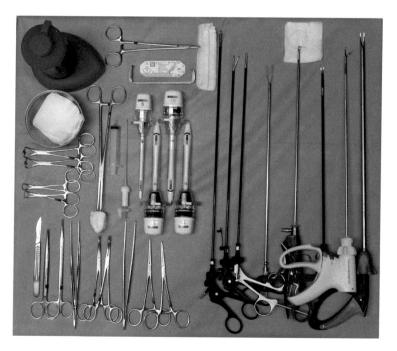

Fig. 6.3 Laparoscopic instrument table

6.2   Pancreatectomy

The bed is placed in reverse Trendelenburg position. First operator stands between patient's legs. Laparoscopic rack is placed behind patient's head (Fig. 6.4).

Specific surgical drapes are used.

Laparotomic Instrument Table Must Be Always Ready for Use

Surgical Steps of Cephalic Pancreatectomy
1. Landmark recognition
2. Epiploon cavity opening
3. Right colic angle mobilization
4. Duodenal and pancreatic mobilization
5. Gastric section
6. Treitz muscle mobilization
7. Digiunal section
8. Isolation and section of choledochus
9. Pancreas isolation and section
10. Retroperitoneal lamina section
11. Specimen extraction
12. Pancreatic-digiunal of pancreatic-gastric anastomosis
13. Gastro-digiunal anastomosis
14. Digiuno-digiunal anastomosis

Surgical Steps of Distal Pancreatectomy
1. Landmark recognition
2. Left colic angle mobilization
3. Short gastric vessel section
4. Isolation of splenic artery (section if needed)
5. Pancreas isolation and section
6. Pancreatectomy (splenectomy if needed)
7. Specimen extraction

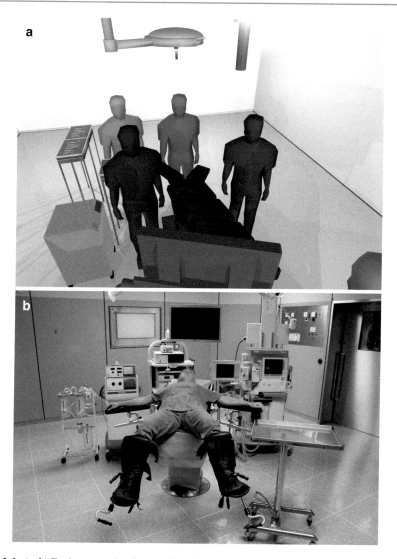

Fig. 6.4 (**a**, **b**) Equipment and patient position during pancreatectomy

Instruments and Cables
- 30 and 5/10 mm laparoscope
- Cold light source cable
- CO_2 pipe and filter
- Monopolar electrocautery
- Patient return electrode (REM)
- Sterile instrument bags
- Bipolar laparotomic forceps
- Monopolar and bipolar electrocautery cables
- Ultrasonic dissector/radiofrequency cables
- Irrigation/suction laparoscopic device
- Bladder catheterization set
- Peridural analgesic catheter and specific set

Laparoscopic Instrument Table (Fig. 6.5)
- Sutures: 2-0 not absorbable braided suture, 2-0 absorbable braided suture, 2-0 braided sutures of different colors, 3-0 barbed suture, 4-0 slowly absorbable suture, and skin wound closure sutures
- Surgical scalpel blade No. 23
- Gauzes
- Laparoscopic gauzes
- Stainless surgical bowl
- Gross-Maier dressing forceps
- Two Bernhard towel forceps
- Veress needle and 10 mL syringe
- Three 10/12 mm trocars
- One/two 5 mm trocars
- Needle holder (different dimensions)
- Two tissue forceps with teeth
- Metzenbaum scissors
- Mayo scissors
- Two Klemmer forceps
- Two Kocher forceps
- Two Backhaus forceps
- Two Farabeuf retractors
- Monopolar crochet hook
- Bipolar laparoscopic forceps
- Ultrasonic dissector/radiofrequency dissector
- Laparoscopic scissors
- Laparoscopic needle holder (2–0, 10 cm long, not absorbable braided must be ready on the instrument)
- Colored (red, white, blue) rubber loops
- Wirsung catheterization

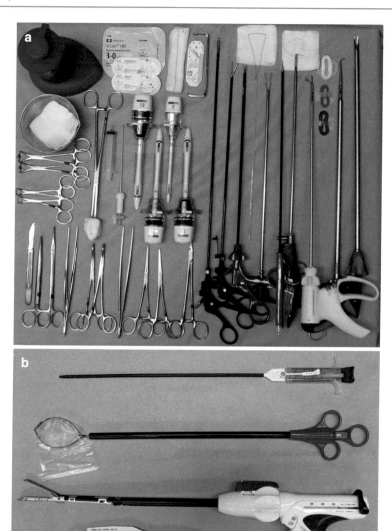

Fig. 6.5 (**a**, **b**) Instrument table

- 5–10 mm clip applier
- Johann forceps without ratchet handle
- 42 cm long Johan forceps without ratchet handle
- Endoloop (2–0 absorbable braided)
- Endo GIA 45/60 mm (blue cartridge for the stomach and for the anastomosis, white cartridge for ileus and the pancreas)
- Laparoscopic 90° forceps with rounded tip
- 15 mm Endobag/wound protector
- Thermos

References

1. Delaitre B, Maignien B (1991) Splenectomy by the laparoscopic approach. Report of a case. Presse Med 20(44):2263, French.
2. Poulin EC, Thibault C (1995) Laparoscopic splenectomy for massive splenomegaly: operative technique and case report. Can J Surg 38(1):69–72.
3. Habermalz B, Sauerland S, Decker G, Delaitre B, Gigot JF, Leandros E, Lechner K, Rhodes M, Silecchia G, Szold A, Targarona E, Torelli P, Neugebauer E (2008) Laparoscopic splenectomy: the clinical practice guidelines of the European Association for Endoscopic Surgery (EAES). Surg Endosc 22(4):821–848.
4. Agresta F, Ansaloni L, Baiocchi GL, Bergamini C, Campanile FC, Carlucci M, Cocorullo G, Corradi A, Franzato B, Lupo M, Mandalà V, Mirabella A, Pernazza G, Piccoli M, Staudacher C, Vettoretto N, Zago M, Lettieri E, Levati A, Pietrini D, Scaglione M, De Masi S, De Placido G, Francucci M, Rasi M, Fingerhut A, Uranüs S, Garattini S (2012) Laparoscopic approach to acute abdomen from the Consensus Development Conference of the Società Italiana di Chirurgia Endoscopica e nuove tecnologie (SICE), Associazione Chirurghi Ospedalieri Italiani (ACOI), Società Italiana di Chirurgia (SIC), Società Italiana di Chirurgia d'Urgenza e del Trauma (SICUT), Società Italiana di Chirurgia nell'Ospedalità Privata (SICOP), and the European Association for Endoscopic Surgery (EAES). Surg Endosc 26(8):2134–2164.
5. Musallam KM, Khalife M, Sfeir PM, Faraj W, Safadi B, Abi Saad GS, Abiad F, Hallal A, Alwan MB, Peyvandi F, Jamali FR (2013) Postoperative outcomes after laparoscopic splenectomy compared with open splenectomy. Ann Surg 257(6):1116–1123.
6. Cabras F, Lazzara F, Bracale U, Andreuccetti J, Pignata G (2014) Single incision laparoscopic splenectomy, technical aspects and feasibility considerations. Wideochir Inne Tech Maloinwazyjne 9(4):632–633.
7. Mehrabi A, Hafezi M, Arvin J, Esmaeilzadeh M, Garoussi C, Emami G, Kössler-Ebs J, Müller-Stich BP, Büchler MW, Hackert T, Diener MK (2015) A systematic review and meta-analysis of laparoscopic versus open distal pancreatectomy for benign and malignant lesions of the pancreas: it's time to randomize. Surgery 157(1):45–55.
8. Yao D, Wu S, Tian Y, Fan Y, Kong J, Li Y (2014) Transumbilical single-incision laparoscopic distal pancreatectomy: primary experience and review of the English literature. World J Surg 38(5):1196–1204.
9. Bracale U, Lazzara F, Andreuccetti J, Stabilini C, Pignata G (2014) Single-access laparoscopic subtotal spleno-pancreatectomy for pancreatic adenocarcinoma. Minim Invasive Ther Allied Technol 23(2):106–109.

Bariatric Surgery

7

Jacopo Andreuccetti, Fabrizio Lazzara, Lidija Ristovich, Michele Lever, and Giusto Pignata

The advent of laparoscopy in the early 1990s has changed the scenario of bariatric surgery by encouraging the spread of certain procedures based on greater acceptance (compliance) of the intervention in a lot of obese patients.

Bariatric surgery, also for the considerable extension of this global disease (globesity), is the branch of surgery in greater and more rapid expansion [1].

In recent years, bariatric surgery is increasingly considered a metabolic surgery. In fact, in the literature, more and more surgical treatment of obesity is related to the treatment of diabetes [2].

There is already irrefutable evidence of experimental and clinical remission of diabetes, more or less immediate and more or less important in the various bariatric surgeries [3–6].

The laparoscopic procedures for obesity can be restrictive or malabsorptive [7].

With restrictive approach, we obtain a reduction of stomach capacity to contain food and therefore food intake. The patient loses weight because the different restrictive surgery induces early satiety.

In other field, malabsorptive interventions confer the ability to reduce the capacity of absorption of food. This type of intervention is most effective in severe obesity because weight loss is not directly related to the caloric intake.

The most commonly performed procedure in the world was Roux-en-Y gastric bypass, followed by sleeve gastrectomy, with significant differences between countries. In fact, in the United States, the sleeve gastrectomy represents the most performed procedure [7].

J. Andreuccetti (✉) • L. Ristovich • M. Lever • G. Pignata
Department of General Surgery, "San Camillo" Hospital, Trento, Italy

Department of General Surgery, Villa Igea Clinic, Acqui Terme, Italy
e-mail: giustopignata@gmail.com; jacopo.andreuccetti@gmail.com

F. Lazzara
Department of General Surgery, Villa Igea Clinic, Acqui Terme, Alessandria, Italy
e-mail: f.lazzara@gmail.com

© Springer International Publishing Switzerland 2016
G. Pignata et al. (eds.), *Laparoscopic Surgery: Key Points, Operating Room Setup and Equipment*, DOI 10.1007/978-3-319-24427-3_7

All these operations can be performed laparoscopically and currently this approach is considered the "gold standard" for obese patients.

7.1 Sleeve Gastrectomy

The bed is placed in reverse Trendelenburg position. First operator stands between patient's legs. Laparoscopic rack is placed behind patient's head. (Fig. 7.1)
Specific surgical drapes are used.

Surgical Steps
1. Landmark recognition
2. Epiploon cavity opening
3. Freeing of long gastric curve
4. Gastric sleeve calibration
5. Gastric transection
6. Suture line reinforcement
7. Suture line check
8. Specimen extraction

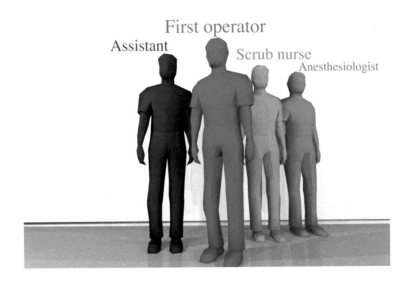

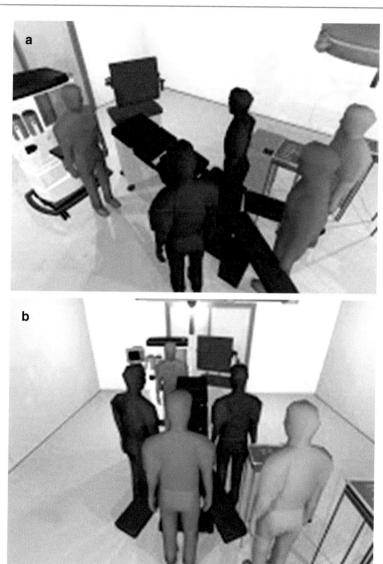

Fig. 7.1 (**a, b, c**) Equipment and patient position during bariatric surgery

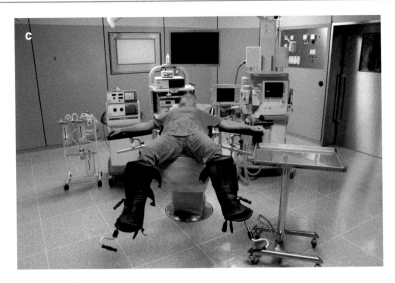

Fig. 7.1 (continued)

Instruments and Cables (Fig. 7.2 a, b)
- 30, 5, or 10 mm laparoscope
- Cold light source cable
- CO_2 pipe and filter
- Monopolar electrocautery
- Patient return electrode (REM)
- Two sterile instrument bags
- Bipolar laparotomic forceps
- Monopolar and bipolar electrocautery cables
- Ultrasonic/radiofrequency cables (bariatric handle)
- Bladder catheterization set
- 56 Fr Maloney probe
- Methylene blue, 60 mL syringe

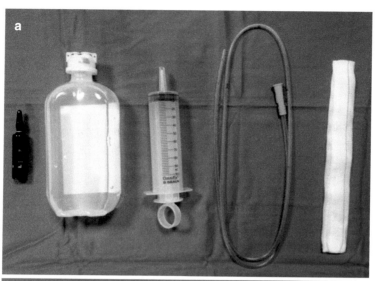

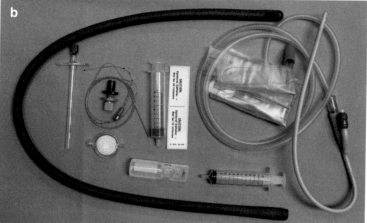

Fig. 7.2 (a–c) Instrument table

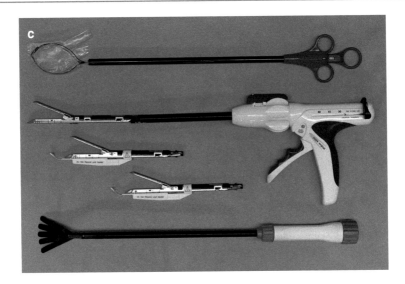

Fig. 7.2 (continued)

Laparoscopic Instrument Table (Fig. 7.2 c)
- Sutures: 3-0 braided slowly absorbable suture and skin wound closure sutures
- Surgical scalpel blade No. 23
- Gauzes
- Laparoscopic gauzes
- Stainless surgical bowl
- Gross-Maier dressing forceps
- Two Bernhard towel forceps
- Veress needle and 10 mL syringe
- Three 10–12 mm trocars
- One 5 mm trocar
- Two needle holder (different dimensions)
- Two tissue forceps with teeth
- Anatomical thumb forceps
- Metzenbaum scissors
- Mayo scissors
- Two Klemmer forceps
- Two Kocher forceps
- Two Backhaus forceps

- Two Farabeuf retractors
- Two Middeldorph retractors
- Two Langenbeck retractors
- Bipolar laparoscopic forceps
- Laparoscopic scissors
- Laparoscopic needle holder (2–0, 10 cm long, not absorbable braided must be ready on the instrument)
- 5–10 mm Endo Retract
- 5–10 mm clip applier
- Two Johann forceps without ratchet handle
- 42 cm long Johann forceps without ratchet handle
- Ultrasonic/radiofrequency dissector (bariatric handle)
- Endo GIA 45/60 mm (green cartridge)
- 15 mm Endobag
- Thermos

7.2   Gastric Bypass: Duodenal Switch

The bed is placed in reverse Trendelenburg position. First operator stands between patient's legs. Laparoscopic rack is placed behind patient's head.
    Specific surgical drapes are used.

Surgical Steps
1. Landmark recognition
2. Digiunal loop measuring
3. Preparation, sectioning, and stitching of different colors on afferent and efferent loop
4. Digiuno-digiunal anastomosis
5. Pars flaccida opening
6. Gastric fundus freeing
7. Gastric section
8. Gastro-digiunal anastomosis
9. Anastomosis check

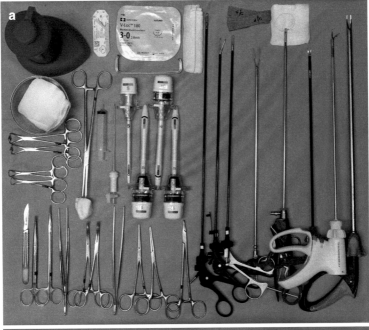

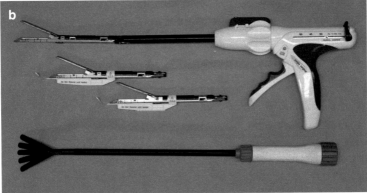

Fig. 7.3 (**a**, **b**) Instrument table

Instruments and Cables
- 30, 5, or 10 mm laparoscope
- Cold light source cable
- CO_2 pipe and filter
- Monopolar electrocautery
- Patient return electrode (REM)
- Two sterile instrument bags

- Bipolar laparotomic forceps
- Monopolar and bipolar electrocautery cables
- Ultrasonic/radiofrequency cables (bariatric handle)
- Bladder catheterization set
- Methylene blue, 60 mL syringe

Laparoscopic Instrument Table (Fig. 7.3 a, b)
- Sutures: 2-0 braided not absorbable suture, 2-0 braided absorbable suture, 2-0 braided suture of different color, 3–0 barbed slowly absorbable suture, and skin wound closure sutures.
- Surgical scalpel blade No. 23
- Gauzes
- Laparoscopic gauzes
- Stainless surgical bowl
- 50 mm sterile tissue band with a sign per centimeter
- Gross-Maier dressing forceps
- Two Bernhard towel forceps
- Veress needle and 10 mL syringe
- Three 10–12 mm trocars
- One 5 mm trocar
- Needle holder
- Two tissue forceps with teeth
- Anatomical thumb forceps
- Metzenbaum scissors
- Mayo scissors
- Two Klemmer forceps
- Two Kocher forceps
- Two Backhaus forceps
- Two Farabeuf retractors
- Bipolar laparoscopic forceps
- Laparoscopic scissors
- Laparoscopic needle holder (2–0, 10 cm long, not absorbable braided must be ready on the instrument)
- 5–10 mm Endo Retract
- 5–10 mm clip applier
- Two Johann forceps without ratchet handle
- 42 cm long Johann forceps without ratchet handle
- Ultrasonic/radiofrequency dissector (bariatric handle)
- Endo GIA 45/60 mm
- Thermos

References

1. National Clinical Guideline Centre (UK) (2014) Obesity: identification, assessment and management of overweight and obesity in children, young people and adults: partial update of CG43. National Institute for Health and Care Excellence (UK), London
2. Scopinaro N (2014) Bariatric metabolic surgery. Rozhl Chir 93(8):404–415
3. Lukas N, Franklin J, Lee CM, Taylor CJ, Martin DJ, Kormas N, Caterson ID, Markovic TP (2014) The efficacy of bariatric surgery performed in the public sector for obese patients with comorbid conditions. Med J Aust 201(4):218–222
4. Ryan D, Heaner M (2014) Guidelines (2013) for managing overweight and obesity in adults. Preface to the full report. Obesity (Silver Spring) 22(Suppl 2):S1–S3
5. Jensen MD, Ryan DH (2014) New obesity guidelines: promise and potential. JAMA 311(1):23–24. doi:10.1001/jama.2013.282546, No abstract available
6. Busetto L, Dixon J, De Luca M, Pories W, Shikora S, Angrisani L (2014) Bariatric surgery. Lancet Diabetes Endocrinol 2(6):448
7. Angrisani L, Santonicola A, Iovino P, Formisano G, Buchwald H, Scopinaro N (2015) Bariatric Surgery Worldwide 2013. Obes Surg. 25(10):1822–1832

Gynecology

8

Francesco Cabras, Fabrizio Lazzara, Lidija Ristovich, Michele Lever, and Giusto Pignata

During the last 40 years, laparoscopy has evolved from a limited gynecologic surgical procedure, used only for diagnosis and tubal ligations, to a major surgical tool operation.

For many gynecologic procedures, such as removal of an ectopic pregnancy, treatment of endometriosis, ovarian cystectomy, and myomectomy, laparoscopy has become the treatment of choice.

Compared with laparotomy, many studies have shown laparoscopy to be safer, to be less expensive, and with shorter recovery time. The advantages of the laparoscopic approach for other procedures, including hysterectomy, sacral colpopexy, and the staging and treatment of gynecologic cancers, continue to broaden [1].

In this oncological view, there are also indications, in skilled hands, to extended lymphadenectomy. In fact, apart from cervical and vaginal cancers that are staged by clinical examination, most gynecological cancers are staged surgically. Pelvic and para-aortic lymphadenectomy offers not only accurate staging information that helps to determine patients' prognosis and hence their treatment plan, but it may also provide a therapeutic effect under certain circumstances. In the past, such procedures required a big laparotomy incision [2].

Laparoscopic techniques have also continued to evolve, primarily as a result of technological advances. In addition, technology has resulted in the development of

F. Cabras (✉)
Department of General Surgery, Colo-Rectal Clinic, "Monserrato Hospital"
University of Cagliari, Cagliari, Italy
e-mail: francescocabras.1@gmail.com

F. Lazzara
Department of General Surgery, Villa Igea Clinic, Acqui Terme, Alessandria, Italy
e-mail: f.lazzara@gmail.com

L. Ristovich • M. Lever • G. Pignata
Department of General Surgery, "San Camillo" Hospital, Trento, Italy
e-mail: giustopignata@gmail.com

© Springer International Publishing Switzerland 2016
G. Pignata et al. (eds.), *Laparoscopic Surgery: Key Points, Operating Room Setup and Equipment*, DOI 10.1007/978-3-319-24427-3_8

robotically assisted laparoscopy and most recently single-port laparoscopy. The relative advantages and disadvantages of these new approaches compared with traditional laparoscopy, as well as their indications, remain to be determined in many cases.

Single-incision laparoscopic surgery (SILS) refers to performing laparoscopy through a single incision. This approach is also referred to as single-access surgery (SAS), single-port surgery (SPS), single-port access (SPA), single-port laparoscopy (SPL), and one-port umbilical surgery (OPUS). Gynecologists have performed SILS for decades, using a 10 mm operating laparoscopes to perform diagnostic laparoscopy and tubal ligations.

The potential benefit of SILS could be a decreased pain, improved cosmetics, and a reduced morbidity associated with port placement.

The major disadvantages of SILS are the lack of triangulation. Articulating instruments are being developed to improve maneuverability; however, these tools have yet to be in common use.

Few gynecologists use the SILS approach because these disadvantages clearly outweigh the potential advantages [3, 4].

Another innovative procedure is the natural orifice transluminal surgery (NOTES). It is an approach that uses an endoscope to access the abdominal cavity through existing body openings, most notably the mouth, rectum, and vagina. This technique combines endoscopic and laparoscopic techniques and can be useful for diagnosis and treatment.

From a historical perspective, gynecologists have reported using NOTES in the form of transvaginal laparoscopy for diagnostic purposes and to perform tubal ligations [5]. Modern NOTES uses a flexible endoscope to access the peritoneal cavity by creating an incision in the stomach or colon.

However, the ability to perform complex operative procedures has so far been limited, and the complication rate, compared to traditional laparoscopy, remains uncertain.

8.1   Hysterectomy

The bed is placed in Trendelenburg position. The patient lies supine, with arms along the body and legs on leg holders. A shoulder holder is needed. Laparoscopic rack is placed at the feet (Fig. 8.1 a, b).

Specific surgical drapes are used.

Laparotomic Instrument Table Must Be Always Ready for Use.

Myomectomy Surgical Steps
1. Uterine cannulation
2. Landmark recognition
3. Myoma enucleation
4. Hemostasis and suture if needed
5. Myoma morcellation or extraction

Hysterectomy Surgical Steps
1. Uterine cannulation
2. Landmark recognition
3. Coagulation and section of round ligament
4. Coagulation and section of utero-ovaric ligament
5. Coagulation and section of large ligament
6. Coagulation and section of uterosacral ligament
7. Coagulation and section of uterine vessels
8. Uterovesical freeing
9. Section of the vagina
10. Uterine morcellation or extraction, vaginal suturing

Ovarian Cyst Excision Surgical Steps
1. Uterine cannulation if needed
2. Landmark recognition
3. Cyst enucleation
4. Hemostasis and suture if needed
5. Cyst extraction

Instruments and Cables
- 30 and 5/10 mm laparoscope
- Cold light source cable
- CO_2 pipe and filter
- Monopolar electrocautery
- Patient return electrode (REM)
- Two sterile instrument bags
- Monopolar and bipolar electrocautery cables
- Ultrasonic dissector/radiofrequency dissector and cables
- Irrigation/suction laparoscopic device
- Bladder catheterization set

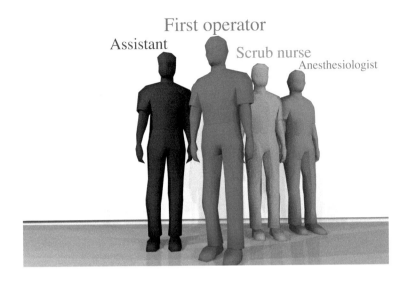

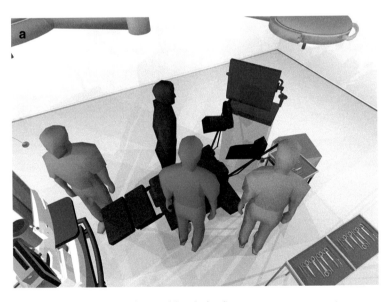

Fig. 8.1 (**a**, **b**) Equipment and patient position during hysterectomy or myomectomy

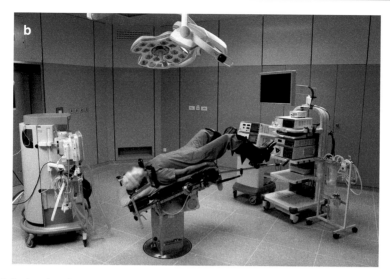

Fig. 8.1 (continued)

Uterine Neck Cannulation (Fig. 8.2a)
- Uterine manipulator set
- Vaginal retractors
- Two Pozzi forceps (for uterine neck)
- Hegar dilatators
- Speculum

Vaginal Instrument Table (Fig. 8.2c)
- Sutures: 0 braided absorbable suture and skin wound closure sutures
- Anterior retractor
- Posterior retractor
- Two Breisky retractors
- Surgical scalpel blade No. 23
- Mayo scissors
- Mayo scissors (bigger)
- Metzenbaum scissors
- Two 18–20 cm long tissue forceps with teeth
- Two anatomical thumb forceps
- Two Debakey forceps
- Four Klemmer forceps

- Four mosquito Kelly forceps
- Four Kocher forceps
- Two 20 cm Kocher forceps
- Two Faure forceps ring tip forceps
- Two Pozzi forceps
- Needle holder

Laparoscopic Instrument Table (Fig. 8.2b)
- Sutures: 2-0 absorbable braided suture, 3-0 braided fast absorbable suture, 3-0 braided slowly absorbable suture and skin wound closure sutures
- Surgical scalpel blade No. 23
- Gauzes
- Laparoscopic gauzes
- Stainless surgical bowl
- Gross-Maier dressing forceps
- Two Bernhard towel forceps
- Veress needle and 10 mL syringe
- Two 10/12 mm trocars
- Two 5 mm trocar
- Uterine morcellator
- Two needle holders (different dimensions)
- Anatomic thumb forceps
- Two tissue forceps with teeth
- Metzenbaum scissors
- Mayo scissors
- Two Klemmer forceps
- Two Kocher forceps
- Two Backhaus forceps
- Two Farabeuf retractors
- Bipolar laparoscopic forceps
- Laparoscopic scissors
- Laparoscopic needle holder (2–0, 10 cm long, not absorbable braided must be ready on the instrument)
- Two Johann forceps without ratchet handle
- Two Manhes forceps
- Crocodile tip forceps
- Thermos

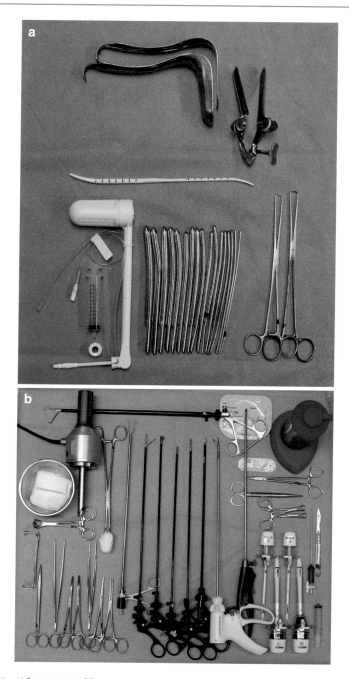

Fig. 8.2 (a–c) Instrument table

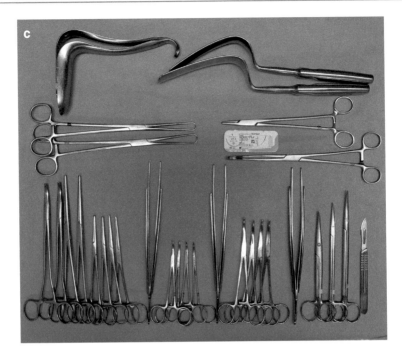

Fig. 8.2 (continued)

8.2   Retroperitoneal Lymphadenectomy

The bed is placed in standard position with shoulder holders. The patient lies in supine position with arms along the body. Laparoscopic rack is placed on the right side and eventually on the left side (Fig. 8.3a, b, Fig. 8.4).

Specific surgical drapes are used.

Laparotomic Instrument Table Must Be Always Ready for Use.

Surgical Steps
1. Landmark recognition
2. Mesenteric root incision
3. Right colon and small bowel mobilization
4. Right renal vein isolation
5. Caval vein and aorta isolation
6. Right gonadic vein section
7. Right ureter isolation
8. Right common iliac vessels isolation
9. Paracaval lymph node excision
10. Left colon mobilization
11. Left ureter isolation
12. Inferior mesenteric artery isolation and section
13. Left renal vein isolation
14. Left gonadic vein section
15. Aortocaval and para-aortic lymph node excision
16. Left common iliac vessel isolation

Instruments and Cables
- 30 and 5/10 mm laparoscope
- Cold light source cable
- CO_2 pipe and filter
- Monopolar electrocautery
- Patient return electrode (REM)
- Two sterile instrument bags
- Bipolar laparotomic forceps
- Monopolar and bipolar electrocautery cables
- Ultrasonic/radiofrequency cables
- Irrigation/suction laparoscopic device
- Bladder catheterization set
- Peridural analgesic catheter and specific set

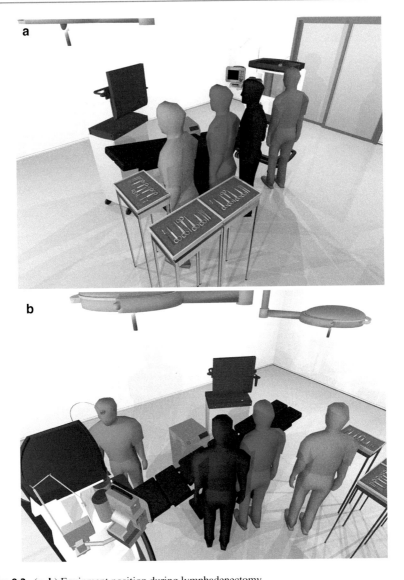

Fig. 8.3 (**a**, **b**) Equipment position during lymphadenectomy

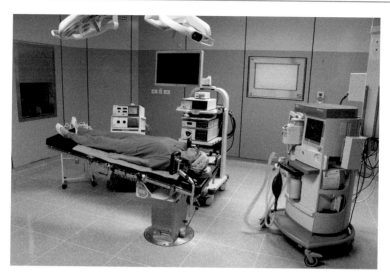

Fig. 8.4   Patient position

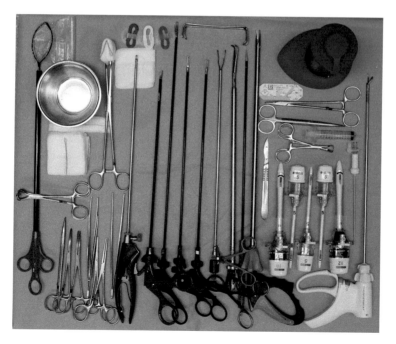

Fig. 8.5   Instrument table

Laparoscopic Instrument Table (Fig. 8.5)

- Sutures: 5-0 or 6-0 monofilament not absorbable sutures with vascular needle and skin wound closure sutures
- Surgical scalpel blade No. 23
- Gauzes
- Laparoscopic gauzes
- Stainless surgical bowl
- Gross-Maier dressing forceps
- Two Bernhard towel forceps
- Veress needle and 10 mL syringe
- 2–3 10/12 mm trocars
- 4–3 5 mm trocars
- One needle holder
- Two tissue forceps with teeth
- Anatomical thumb forceps
- Metzenbaum scissors
- Mayo scissors
- Two Klemmer forceps
- Two Kocher forceps
- Two Backhaus forceps
- Two Farabeuf retractors
- Bipolar laparoscopic forceps
- Ultrasonic dissector/radiofrequency dissector
- Laparoscopic scissors
- Monopolar Crochet hook
- Laparoscopic needle holder (5–0, 10 cm long, not absorbable monofilament suture must be ready on the instrument)
- 5–10 mm clip applier
- Two Johann forceps without ratchet handle
- 42 cm long Johann forceps without ratchet handle
- 5–10 mm Endo Retract
- Laparoscopic 90° forceps with rounded tip
- Colored (red, yellow, blue) rubber loops
- 10 mm Endobag
- Thermos

References

1. Walker JL, Piedmonte MR, Spirtos NM, Eisenkop SM, Schlaerth JB, Mannel RS et al (2012) Recurrence and survival after random assignment to laparoscopy versus laparotomy for comprehensive surgical staging of uterine cancer: Gynecologic Oncology Group LAP2 Study. J Clin Oncol 30(7):695–700
2. Tse KY, Ngan HY (2015) The role of laparoscopy in staging of different gynaecological cancers. Best Pract Res Clin Obstet Gynaecol. pii:S1521-6934(15)
3. Bradford LS, Boruta DM (2013) Laparoendoscopic single-site surgery in gynecology: a review of the literature, tools, and techniques. Obstet Gynecol Surv 68(4):295–304
4. Rosati M, Bosev D, Thiella R, Capobianco F, Bracale U, Azioni G (2010) Single port laparoscopically assisted hysterectomy with the TriPort system. A case report and review of the literature. Ann Ital Chir 81(3):221–225
5. Abarbanel AR (1955) Transvaginal pelvioscopy (peritoneoscopy); a simplified and safe technic as an office procedure. Am J Surg 90(1):122–128